Recovering Together:
Building Resiliency After
Acute Neurological Illness

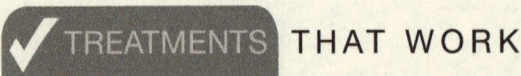

✔ TREATMENTS THAT WORK

Recovering Together: Building Resiliency After Acute Neurological Illness

CLINICIAN GUIDE

ANA-MARIA VRANCEANU

VICTORIA A. GRUNBERG

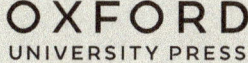

OXFORD
UNIVERSITY PRESS

OXFORD
UNIVERSITY PRESS

Oxford University Press is a department of the University of Oxford.
It furthers the University's objective of excellence in research, scholarship,
and education by publishing worldwide. Oxford is a registered trade mark of
Oxford University Press in the UK and certain other countries.

Published in the United States of America by Oxford University Press
198 Madison Avenue, New York, NY 10016, United States of America.

CIP data is on file at the Library of Congress

ISBN 978–0–19–769390–2

DOI: 10.1093/med-psych/9780197693902.001.0001

Printed by Marquis Book Printing, Canada

The manufacturer's authorized representative in the EU for product safety is
Oxford University Press España S.A., Parque Empresarial San Fernando de Henares,
Avenida de Castilla, 2 – 28830 Madrid (www.oup.es/en).

MIX
Paper | Supporting
responsible forestry
FSC
www.fsc.org   FSC® C103567

BEHAVIORAL MEDICINE PROGRAMS

People who are at risk for or living with a medical illness often face difficult challenges engaging in behavior changes that might be necessary to optimize their health. These challenges can include overcoming barriers to care, managing psychological distress (e.g., depression, anxiety), and coping with changes in how they interact with friends, family, or community. People with a medical illness often need to make behavioral changes to enhance their health such as taking medications, managing multiple medical appointments, increasing exercise, reducing substance intake, changing one's diet, participating in rehabilitation, managing side effects of treatments or new symptoms. In addition to the medical component, a huge part of managing illness and prevention is the human component.

Behavioral medicine interventions, or those that address the psychological and behavioral component of medical care, are critical for the success of any medical treatment, prevention agent, or cure. However, participating in such interventions often takes a lot of time, energy, and effort over and above the effort needed to just keep up with medical appointments and other parts of their life. Adding this component can be challenging on top of managing their illness, day, job, family, and other responsibilities.

A stumbling block for clinicians is the accessibility of newly developed evidence-based behavioral medicine interventions. This series, *Treatments That Work: Behavioral Medicine Programs*, addresses this by presenting the latest and most effective interventions for particular problems in user-friendly language. To be included in this series, each program must display the highest standards of evidence available, as determined by a scientific advisory board. The manuals and workbooks in this series contain detailed step-by-step procedures for assessing and treating specific problems and diagnoses. But this series also goes beyond the books and manuals by providing ancillary materials that will approximate the supervisory process in assisting practitioners to implement these procedures in their practice.

Acute neurological illnesses (ANI; e.g., stroke, traumatic brain injury, benign brain tumor) are common and often traumatic for patients and the family and friends who support them (caregivers). About 20% to 40% of patients and caregivers experience symptoms of emotional distress (depression, anxiety, posttraumatic stress) early after hospitalization. This early distress is interdependent between patients and caregivers and, if untreated, can become chronic and negatively impact the patient's recovery, the caregiver's ability to provide care to the patient, and the quality of life for both.

The Recovering Together program aims to prevent chronic emotional distress among patients who experienced an ANI and their caregivers (together called a dyad). This six-session, seven-module (the dyad will choose which six of the seven sessions to use), dyadic program (patient and caregiver are treated together) seeks to promote individual and interpersonal resiliency. It integrates skills from evidence-based interventions including mindfulness-based stress reduction, cognitive behavioral therapy, dialectical behavior therapy, and positive psychology approaches. Recovering Together is a flexible intervention that can be implemented in medical (e.g., intensive care unit), virtual (via live video), or outpatient mental health settings. The processes and skills presented here stem from treatments that have decades of empirical support. However, these skills are simplified and delivered with pictorials and simple language to facilitate uptake within the context of an ANI.

This Clinician Guide is intended to be used by clinicians who are familiar with second- and third-wave cognitive behavioral therapies. Unique challenges of an ANI include the acuity of the event, unexpected and heterogeneous diagnoses and prognosis, and impact on caregivers. Recovering Together helps address these issues by being flexible (offered shortly after the event in the medical setting or at discharge), tailored (suitable for different ANI diagnoses and mental health symptoms), and dyadic (patient and caregiver are treated together). This program is an invaluable resource for practitioners who wish to effectively and efficiently prevent chronic distress and enhance interpersonal processes among patients who experienced an ANI and their caregivers.

Steven A. Safren, Editor-in-Chief
David H. Barlow, Editor-in-Chief
Treatments That Work: Behavioral Medicine Programs

Contents

Introductory Information for Clinicians

Background Information and Purpose of This Program

Recovering Together is a six-session, seven-module skills-based resiliency intervention for patients with acute neurological illnesses (ANIs) and their caregivers (i.e., family member or friend providing care; together, called "dyads"). ANIs (e.g., stroke/hemorrhage, brain aneurysm, brain tumors or masses, and traumatic brain injuries) are often sudden and life-threatening, thereby requiring emergency care (Hirtz et al., 2007). This experience can be traumatic both for patients and their caregivers, giving rise to long-term psychiatric sequelae (Denno et al., 2013). In fact, 20% to 40% of ANI patients and their caregivers experience clinically significant emotional distress (i.e., depression, anxiety, and posttraumatic stress) during hospitalization (Denno et al., 2013). After hospital discharge, emotional distress can become chronic and interfere with recovery and quality of life (Ayerbe et al., 2013).

Recovering Together is a transdiagnostic program, addressing the comorbidity of depression, anxiety, and posttraumatic stress (PTS). It is the first dyadic intervention (treating patient and caregiver together) for preventing chronic emotional distress in patients with ANIs and their caregivers. It was iteratively developed and optimized with feedback from patients, caregivers, and medical teams (Vranceanu et al., 2020, 2022).

Recovering Together focuses on promoting individual and interpersonal resiliency among patients and caregivers. It integrates evidence-based approaches including mindfulness, cognitive behavioral therapy (CBT), and dialectical behavior therapy (DBT). It teaches mindfulness skills (e.g., deep breathing, present moment awareness), coping skills (e.g., dialectics, meaning-making, adaptive thinking), and interpersonal skills (e.g., communication, coping with role changes). In the first few sessions, dyads process their experience and learn diaphragmatic breathing, mindfulness, and dialectics. The subsequent four sessions are tailored to the dyad's specific challenges, needs, and concerns (Vranceanu et al., 2020, 2022). During these sessions, dyads learn how to restructure their thoughts, communicate effectively, accept what they cannot change, engage in valued activities, and/or reflect on their experience.

As presented in Table I.1: Recovering Together Session Content (located near the end of this Introduction), to promote individualized care, the dyad and clinician together choose the next four sessions out of five available sessions. However, the dyad has access to all sessions (via the Recovering Together Patient and Caregiver Workbook [hereafter referred to as "the Workbook"]) and the supplemental website, which can be accessed by searching for this book's title on the Oxford Academic platform at academic.oup.com. The website includes session content, skills, and additional materials (e.g., recordings, videos) to facilitate practice. The dyad is encouraged to practice skills between sessions (referred to as the "Prescription for Recovery"). The clinician checks in each session to help problem-solve barriers to home practice.

Recovering Together can be delivered across different settings. The first one or two sessions typically occur during hospitalization at bedside in a medical setting, such as the Neuroscience Intensive Care Unit (Neuro-ICU). The following four or five sessions are typically delivered virtually (over secure live video) after discharge. Recovering Together can also be delivered in rehabilitative settings or entirely virtually. The format is flexible given the various trajectories of patients with ANI and the challenges of scheduling a time when both the patient and caregiver are available. When possible, it is helpful for the first session to be in person or for the clinician to meet the dyad prior to discharge because it helps build rapport. However, the program is meant to be flexible and is effective across medical, rehabilitative, home, and virtual settings. Dyad members can be in the same or different locations (patient at bedside; caregiver over live video). Because sessions often take place in the medical setting shortly after admission, sessions can be brief, skills are simplified, and mindfulness and dialectics skills are integrated throughout the program.

Table I.1 Recovering Together Session Content

Session Number and Title	When to Deliver the Session	Skills Covered in the Session
1. Staying in the Here and Now	General (Neuro-ICU)	■ Discuss and learn about common challenges for patients and caregivers after ANI. ■ Learn the skill of Deep Breathing to decrease anxiety, panic, or distress. ■ Learn about the three steps of the Mindful Stoplight: Observe, Describe, Act with Awareness. ■ Use the Mindful Stoplight to Stay in the 24-Hour Block. ■ Learn how to practice Mindfulness Meditation. ■ Receive weekly Prescription for Recovery.
2. Coping with Uncertainty	General (Neuro-ICU)	■ Review last session and Prescription for Recovery. ■ Learn the value of Dialectics (seeing both sides). ■ Identify dialectical thoughts and emotions. ■ Practice Hands as Worries skill (i.e., flexibility during times of stress). ■ Receive weekly Prescription for Recovery.
3. Adjusting to Life After an Acute Neurological Illness (ANI)	Specific (after Neuro-ICU)	■ Review last session and Prescription for Recovery. ■ Understand patient and caregiver's stressors. ■ Learn about Identifying the Distress Spiral. ■ Learn about Challenging Unhelpful Thoughts after an ANI. ■ Receive weekly Prescription for Recovery.
4. Navigating Relationships	Specific (after Neuro-ICU)	■ Review last session and Prescription for Recovery ■ Use Mindful Stoplight and Dialectics to identify and adjust to changes after ANI. ■ Learn Effective Communication strategies for having difficult conversations. ■ Practice sharing individual experiences and active listening to better work as a team. ■ Receive weekly Prescription for Recovery.

(Continued)

Table I.1 Continued

Session Number and Title	When to Deliver the Session	Skills Covered in the Session
5. Engaging with Positive Activities	Specific (after Neuro-ICU)	▪ Review prior sessions and Prescription for Recovery. ▪ Learn the value of Behavioral Activation to improve mood. ▪ Discuss the importance of using Social Support. ▪ Practice the skill of setting Daily Goals. ▪ Receive weekly Prescription for Recovery.
6. Managing Fear and Worries	Specific (after Neuro-ICU)	▪ Review prior sessions and Prescription for Recovery. ▪ Use the Mindful Stoplight skill to practice Observing Fear and Worry. ▪ Discuss the importance of Acceptance and Change (Dialectics). ▪ Learn when to practice acceptance and/or make changes. ▪ Receive weekly Prescription for Recovery.
7. Making Meaning	Specific (after Neuro-NICU)	▪ Review prior sessions and Prescription for Recovery. ▪ Learn the value of Making Meaning for recovery. ▪ Practice Making Meaning using reflection questions. ▪ Use Mindful Stoplight and Dialectics to find meaning. ▪ Receive weekly Prescription for Recovery.

Recovering Together is for patients who experienced an ANI. Patients and families are often in shock because of the unexpected nature of the event. Given the acuity of and stress associated with an ANI, it is important for clinicians to build rapport with the dyad. Having a strong therapeutic alliance promotes engagement. We encourage you, as the clinician, to be flexible and tailor the content and skills however you see fit. At times, patients will be sleepy or in pain, so you can make the session shorter or focus on the caregiver. Then, you can revisit the skills in later sessions. We describe the importance of tailoring skills and being flexible in more detail in later chapters.

Recovering Together works well for patients and/or caregivers who endorse clinically significant distress on validated assessments (Hospital Anxiety and Depression Scale [HADS; Zigmond & Snaith, 1983]; Posttraumatic Stress Disorder Checklist for DSM-5 [PCL-5; Blevins et al., 2015]). We encourage clinicians to assess depression, anxiety, and PTS symptoms each week using the HADS and/or PCL-5 (or another measure). You can send the measures over email or have the dyad complete them at the beginning of each session. Regular assessment of symptoms allows you to track progress and tailor the skills to help address specific symptoms.

As noted, Recovery Together is a dyadic intervention. Given the interdependence of stress and coping, its dyadic format can help reduce distress in both members and improve interactions. The caregiver can be any family member or friend (even if they do not live with the patient). Although the caregiver is often a spouse, it does not have to be an intimate partner. The goals are to promote adaptive coping as individuals and a team. It is important for the clinician to prompt both the patient and caregiver to share their experiences. Normalize that this experience impacts each of them and their relationship. Prompt both dyad members to discuss their unique and shared experiences. It is helpful for patients and caregivers to share, listen, and engage in crosstalk during the session. We encourage you to pay attention to their relationship dynamic and promote open communication throughout all sessions.

Disorder or Problem Focus and Diagnostic Criteria

Recovering Together addresses emotional distress (e.g., symptoms of depression, anxiety, and PTS) in the context of an ANI (e.g., status epilepticus, ischemic stroke, brain aneurysm, and traumatic brain injury) that requires hospitalization in a critical care setting (CCS) such as an intensive care unit (ICU) or Neuro-ICU. This program addresses emotional distress for patients, caregivers, and the patient–caregiver dyad. While the program was developed specifically for dyads with an acute brain illness, it can be used across critical care illnesses that are sudden, traumatic, and life-threatening.

Symptoms of depression, anxiety, and PTS are common in this population early after hospitalization and often become chronic, which can negatively impact physical recovery and increase risk for morbidity and mortality. These lasting effects can also occur in patients' caregivers (e.g., family and friends) for years following a loved one's illness. This distress impacts caregivers' and patients' quality of life after hospitalization (Davydow et al., 2012; Wintermann et al., 2016).

Posttraumatic Stress Disorder

Posttraumatic stress disorder (PTSD) is a response to a life-threatening event that continues for at least 4 weeks after the trauma and includes avoidance of trauma reminders, physiological hyperarousal, re-experiencing, and negative cognitions (Yehuda, 2002). Since the acute illness and subsequent hospitalization in a CCS are often sudden and life-threatening, many patients develop PTS symptoms that can transition to PTSD. Caregivers who witness life-threatening chronic critical illness can also develop PTSD (Choi et al., 2016; van Beusekom et al., 2016; van den Born-van Zanten et al., 2016). The prevalence of PTSD in survivors is high and persists over time (Myhren et al., 2010). More than 75% of mixed ICU patients referred for neuropsychological evaluation report at least one stressful in-ICU experience (e.g., nightmares, severe pain, breathing difficulty, or a feeling of suffocation) (Chung et al., 2017). A meta-analysis in 36 unique cohorts of patients surviving critical illness found a pooled prevalence of PTSD of 25% to 44% at 6 months, depending on the severity cutoff used (Parker et al., 2015). At 1-year follow-up, PTSD symptoms are still reported in upwards of 20% of survivors (Parker et al., 2015). Rates of PTSD in caregivers of ICU survivors range between 11.1% and 57.1%, depending on the instrument used and timepoint of assessment (Gries et al., 2010; Petrinec & Martin, 2018; van Beusekom et al., 2016; Wintermann et al., 2016; Zimmerli et al., 2014). These high prevalence rates are corroborated by studies using the PCL-5, which has a high concordance with diagnostic interviews (K. W. Choi et al., 2018). For the purpose of this program, we are using the PCL linked to the ANI and hospitalization for both patients and caregivers.

Depression

In a large multicenter study investigating neuropsychological health after critical illness, the reported prevalence of depression was 37% (Jackson et al., 2014). In patients with no preexisting history of depression, depressive symptoms still occur in nearly 30% at 12 months, and the prevalence is even higher in patients with preexisting depression. At 5 years, prevalence is still nearly 20% in a multicenter cohort study of survivors (Adhikari et al., 2011). Smaller cohorts have a wider range of rates of depression, though they are still significantly higher than the general population prevalence of less than 10% (Jackson et al., 2011; Kessler et al., 2005; Mikkelsen et al., 2012). Similarly, rates of depression in caregivers range between 4.7% and 36% (Gries et al., 2010; Petrinec & Martin, 2018; Siegel et al., 2008; van Beusekom et al., 2016). Some researchers have noted a long-lasting comorbidity between ICU-associated depression and PTSD (Paparrigopoulos et al., 2014). In Recovering Together, we assess and monitor symptoms of depression using the HADS (depression subscale).

Anxiety

Rates of anxiety range from 16% to 24% in long-term survivors of critical care illness, though rates as high as 62% have been reported (Hopkins et al., 2010; Mikkelsen et al., 2012; Myhren et al., 2010). These prevalence rates of anxiety are higher than those in the general population (Kessler et al., 2005). Caregivers experience anxiety with rates similar to those of patients (15% to 25%) (van Beusekom et al., 2016).

Development and Evidence Base of Recovering Together

The development of Recovering Together came from a critical need. As more patients survive their Neuro-ICU stay due to advances in technology and medical care, the long-term psychiatric sequalae associated with the sudden and traumatic onset of the ANI have become increasingly recognized. As noted in the prior section, rates of clinically significant symptoms of anxiety, depression, and PTSD are high among both patients and caregivers, interrelated within dyads, and sustained over time. Prior interventions to support these needs have had less-than-encouraging results. For example, a systematic review and meta-analysis showed the potential for ICU diaries to reduce the risk for depression and anxiety in ICU survivors, but not in caregivers and not for posttraumatic symptoms (Barreto et al., 2019). Unfortunately, only three randomized clinical trials (RCTs), with very small samples, were included in the review, diminishing generalizability. Wade and colleagues (2019) reported on a large, multicenter, cluster RCT of a nurse-led CBT intervention among at-risk ICU survivors that showed no significant reduction in posttraumatic symptom severity 6 months after discharge. White and colleagues (2012) reported on a large stepped-wedge cluster RCT of a nurse-delivered family support intervention for surrogates of critically ill patients from five ICUs and found no effect on improvement in emotional distress when compared with control.

As a result, our psychology team partnered with nurses and critical care doctors to develop an evidence-based solution to address early emotional distress in patients and caregivers. We built on the limitations of prior research and used the National Institutes of Health (NIH) stage model to create Recovering Together. We first conducted qualitative interviews with dyads (patients with an acute brain illness and their caregivers) to understand population needs and barriers and facilitators to participation (McCurley et al., 2019). We also conducted focus groups with nurses and shared our results with the Neuro-ICU leadership (McCurley et al., 2019).

This preliminary qualitative work combined with results from our prospective studies summarized in prior sections supported several content and methodological decisions:

1. It highlighted the need to start the intervention in person at bedside and continue through discharge home or to the rehabilitation setting via secure video.
2. It showed the need for a transdiagnostic intervention that can address the construct of emotional distress rather than only depression, anxiety, or PTS symptoms.
3. Because distress and coping are interdependent between patients and caregivers, we elected to use a dyadic approach to treatment and include the patient and caregivers together in sessions.

4. Rather than developing new skills, we deconstructed existing evidence-based skills and simplified them so that they can be more easily digested by patients with cognitive concerns and dyads in acute distress. We also used mindfulness-based and DBT skills in the early sessions to address the initial stress associated with critical illness, the uncertainty of prognosis, and concerns about each other's well-being, which are key concerns early after hospitalization. We next moved to more cognitive skills in later sessions and after discharge, when the medical situation of the patient was stabilized, and dyads were better able to engage with higher-order skills.
5. Because dyads have heterogeneous presentations with regard to their medical diagnoses, prognoses, life contexts, and emotional distress symptoms, we designed Recovering Together as a tailored intervention that includes flexible modular post-hospitalization sessions that are delivered to meet the unique needs of each dyad.

We next tested Recovering Together in an open pilot study with exit interviews and published a case paper delineating the content of the program and how it was applied to a stroke dyad (Meyers et al., 2020). We iterated the program through a small pilot RCT that informed the current version, which we tested for preliminary efficacy in a single-blind RCT against an educational control (Bannon et al., 2020). This trial showed that participation in Recovering Together was associated with statistically and clinically significant improvement in depression, anxiety, and PTSD over and above control (Bannon et al., 2022). Another large, single-blind RCT is in progress (Vranceanu et al., 2022). Pending positive results from this trial, we will work to implement Recovering Together as part of usual care within ICUs from across the country.

Recovering Together is the first dyadic, modular skills-based intervention aimed at preventing chronic emotional distress in at-risk dyads with an acute brain illness. The program is informed by:

- Theoretical response-shift framework of adaptation to acute illness (successful adaptation implies recalibration of values and life goals) (Barclay-Goddard et al., 2012),
- Family strength vulnerability model (within dyads, relational systems have strengths and weaknesses in how they cope with life events) (Shields et al., 1995),

- Dyadic stress and coping model (coping together with life events is associated with positive adaptation) (Bodenmann et al., 2019), and
- Resiliency theory processes (resiliency is multidimensional and involves multiple factors that foster adaptation) (Southwick et al., 2014).

Informed by these theoretical models, our conceptual model hypothesizes that by teaching both members of the dyads resiliency and interpersonal communication skills, we will be able to decrease emotional distress in dyads.

As previously stated, the skills in this program are evidence-based, drawn systematically from mindfulness, cognitive behavioral, and positive psychology principles. The first two sessions teach concrete skills focused on helping dyads get through the trauma of the hospitalization and focus on self-care. The subsequent four sessions are tailored to the specific needs of each dyad based on specific challenges, sequelae, or concerns identified collaboratively by the clinician and dyad.

Psychotherapy Approaches

Recovering Together integrates skills from several evidence-based interventions, including mindfulness-based stress reduction, DBT, CBT, and positive psychology and acceptance-based approaches. The core components of the program, mindfulness and dialectics, are integrated into nearly every session.

Mindfulness

Mindfulness has been defined as paying attention to the present moment, on purpose and without judgment (Kabat-Zinn, 2003). Mindfulness involves two components: (1) regulating attention to become more aware of experiences (e.g., thoughts, emotions, physical sensations) and (2) embracing openness and nonjudgment to accept experiences as they are, regardless of their positive or negative valence (Kabat-Zinn, 2003). In Recovering Together, we teach mindfulness in multiple ways, including through a Mindful Stoplight metaphor ("Observe, Describe, and Act with Awareness") based on "what skills" of mindfulness in DBT (Linehan

& Wilks, 2015; Rizvi et al., 2013), Staying in the 24-Hour Block, and Mindfulness Meditation. We also use it as a tool to facilitate the skill of Effective Communication between dyad members. For example, we encourage dyad members to Observe and Describe their individual experiences and approach conversations with curiosity and openness.

Dialectics

Dialectics, primarily used in DBT, is both a theoretical stance and a strategy for change (May et al., 2016). The theory notes that reality comprises interrelated and connected worldviews, including opposing and changing forces. Dialectics means that multiple or opposing views can exist at the same time (Rizvi et al., 2013). This technique is beneficial for medical patients who often have multiple emotions and reactions to their sudden hospitalization (e.g., "I'm grateful for the care I received" and "I'm angry that this happened"). In Recovering Together, this skill is key both within and between the members of each dyad. We encourage patient and caregiver to each identify their own dialectical experience as well as how both of their experiences can exist together. For example, caregivers often feel that they should not express their stress (out of fear of making patients more distressed). However, when caregivers acknowledge their own challenges, it allows the patient to support the caregiver—which is often important for the patient's own adjustment. It is important for patients and caregivers to acknowledge their individual dialectics (e.g., sadness, fear, grief, relief) and dyadic dialectics (e.g., patient is worried while caregiver is hopeful, or vice versa). In Recovering Together, we also discuss Acceptance Versus Change (Dialectics). This dialectic is important for this population because it helps them to accept the reality of this event while encouraging them to make positive changes in health behaviors or coping.

Risks and Benefits

Recovering Together has promising benefits. Research indicates that it can help reduce symptoms of depression, anxiety, and PTS among patients and caregivers. The program has also been shown to help improve interactions among patients and caregivers (Vranceanu et al.,

2020). In addition, offering Recovering Together in medical settings helps to normalize distress and increase awareness of and access to psychosocial treatment.

There are no direct physical risks to participating in this program. However, it is possible that sharing thoughts and emotions may be difficult or cause discomfort. It is important to develop a strong therapeutic alliance and tailor treatment to each dyad's needs and presentations. Further, the program can seem time-consuming for some dyads. It is important to provide psychoeducation about how the program can help them manage everyday challenges. We also encourage clinicians to validate all levels of dyad engagement (e.g., attending sessions, practicing skills, completing the program). Given the multiple demands on caregivers and the medical complications of the patient, it is helpful to validate the fact that they are making time for each other and their emotional health.

Alternative Treatments

To date, there are no evidence-based treatments to address symptoms of depression, anxiety, and PTSD among dyads of patients hospitalized for an ANI and their family caregivers. The current usual-care model includes psychiatry consultations for psychotropic medications and referrals for psychotherapy after discharge, and visits with social workers for case management or coordination of care. Patients and caregivers could benefit from individual traditional CBT or mindfulness-based approaches after discharge, particularly when the therapist is skilled in understanding the complexity of the critical care experience. Couples therapy or dyadic therapy can also be useful to work through challenges with communication around role changes and adjustment to survivor and caregiver roles. Studies assessing the efficacy of these approaches are limited.

The Role of Medications

For the Patient

Psychotropic medications are sometimes prescribed to critical care patients. For example, 17% of patients admitted to an ICU were prescribed a new psychotropic medication (Vehviläinen et al., 2021). The majority of medications were antidepressants (61%), antipsychotics, (35%) and anxiolytics (26%) (Hammond et al., 2015; Vehviläinen et al., 2021). After adjusting for injury severity, new psychotropic medication was associated with increased odds of late mortality (Vehviläinen et al., 2021). A recent review of psychotropic drug therapy in ICU patients shows that using psychotropic drugs might increase the risk of drug–drug interactions (e.g., drugs for the management of the physical symptoms of the critical care injury and the psychotropic drug) (Shafiekhani et al., 2018).

Benzodiazepines are generally administered to critically ill patients to achieve a state of deep sedation and amnesia, as well as for their antianxiety effects. They have a hypnotic, anticonvulsant, and muscle relaxant effect that is desirable for selected ICU patients (Devlin & Roberts, 2009). However, side effects such as respiratory suppression, reduced blood pressure, and delirium are common and heightened by drug–drug interactions (Devlin & Roberts, 2009; Fraser et al., 2013; Thomason et al., 2005). Typically, it is recommended that use of benzodiazepines should be limited in patients with head trauma, intracranial hemorrhages, or epilepsy to prevent increase of intracranial pressure. If benzodiazepines are required, they should be prescribed for the shortest amount of time possible and at the lower dose (Barr et al., 2013). Alpha-2 agonists are preferred over benzodiazepines for inducing sedation because they can prevent delirium in ICU settings. The incidence of adverse events is high for propofol, and ketamine, while favorable for rapid sequence intubation, causes psychological complications in a dose-dependent manner. Antipsychotics are not recommended, particularly in patients prone to arrhythmias. Generally, it is recommended to wait to prescribe antidepressants until the patient is in a stable condition, to avoid side effects (Kelly et al., 2017).

For the Caregiver

Medications can also be helpful for caregivers. Although caregivers are not considered "patients" in our current health care systems, it would be important for the medical team to encourage psychopharmacological consultations when high caregiver distress is noted.

Each session is 30 to 45 minutes. The sessions are delivered weekly, although early sessions can be held more frequently (within a week) if the dyad prefers to meet in person before discharge. All sessions follow the same format:

1. Check in and review home practice,
2. Set agenda,
3. Review skills and practice in session, and
4. Discuss Prescription for Recovery (home practice plan over next week).

As stressed multiple times above, we encourage you to tailor the content and skills to the dyad's needs.

Table I.1, "Recovering Together Session Content," details each session, including the session numbers and titles, when to deliver the session, and skills covered. Sessions 1 and 2 are key components of the program and therefore are always delivered. Then, in collaboration with the clinician, the dyads choose four of the five remaining sessions. These sessions should be delivered in chronological order. Therefore, the final session is either Session 6 or 7 (depending on which sessions they choose). Although they can pick any of the sessions, Sessions 3, 4, and 7 are frequently chosen. Dyads usually choose between Sessions 5 and 6 depending on whether they present with more depressive or anxiety symptoms. Session 5, "Engaging with Positive Activities," works well for depression and Session 6, "Managing Fear and Worries," works well for anxiety.

Use of the Corresponding Workbook

Both dyad members should receive their own Workbook. The Clinician Guide directly corresponds with the Workbook (same headings and subheadings). The clinician should provide the dyad with their Workbooks in Session 1. They should continue to bring the Workbook to each session. It is designed to facilitate practice in and out of session. It includes exercises that they can complete. This program's supplemental website offers additional home practice opportunities (videos, recordings) and can be accessed by searching for this book's title on the Oxford Academic platform at academic.oup.com. Clinicians should orient the dyad to the website (in addition to the Workbook) during Session 1.

Given that the patients experienced a recent stroke or brain illness or other neurological event, the illustrations in the Workbook will help them master the information. Clinicians should point out the icons/graphics that correspond to each skill. The pictorial representations of skills are presented at the beginning of each session. The skills from prior sessions are also included to remind the patient and caregiver to practice. There is also a Prescription for Recovery at the end of each session to help dyads plan when they will practice the skills for the week. Home practice is an important way for dyads to learn and apply the skills in everyday life.

CHAPTER 1

Session 1: Staying in the Here and Now

(Corresponds to Session 1 of the Workbook)

Materials

- Clinician Guide and Workbooks
- Pens

Outline of Session 1

Session 1 Goals

Preparing for Session 1

  Setting and Context

  - Recommendations for Clinicians
  - Logistics for Delivery
  - Assessment and Chart Review (administer and/or review measures of depression, anxiety, and posttraumatic stress for each dyad member)

Session 1

  - Introductions and Rapport-Building
  - Overview and Rationale of Program

Agenda

Education

Skills (Teach and Practice)

  - Deep Breathing
  - Mindful Stoplight
  - Staying in the 24-Hour Block
  - Mindfulness Meditation

Session 1 Summary

Prescription for Recovery (Home Practice)

Schedule Next Session

1. Make a meaningful connection with the patient and their caregiver. A strong therapeutic alliance is key for participation and retention. Show compassion, curiosity, care, and genuine interest in learning about them as individuals and a team.

2. Assess the readiness and interest of each dyad member. They often have different levels of emotional distress and buy-in. Encourage them to meet each other where they are and explain that their participation demonstrates their support for each other.

3. It is often the case that the caregiver will prioritize care for the patient because they are experiencing the acute illness. It is important to ensure that both the patient and caregiver understand that their emotional recovery is interdependent; by practicing skills and caring for themselves, they help the other person recover.

4. Teach skills in a way that shows their applicability to everyday life. Practice them during the session and ensure that dyads understand how to use them (rather than only as abstract concepts). Mindfulness is foundational to this program, so make sure they understand the different ways they can use it.

Preparing for Session 1

Setting and Context

Session 1 occurs at the bedside in the Neurosciences Intensive Care Unit (Neuro-ICU) or an Intensive Care Unit (ICU). Many patients and families are admitted to the ICU unexpectedly. During hospitalization, they worry about the patient's survival and outcomes, the impact on the family, and how they will adjust to a new normal. Families are under extreme stress, which can interfere with their health behaviors (sleep, eating), judgment and decision-making, and communication. This experience places them at risk for chronic emotional distress, which is why early intervention is vital.

Recommendations for Clinicians

Given this unique context, we have important recommendations for you:

1. Keep the session brief (~30 minutes). Patients receive 24-hour multidisciplinary care and can be sleepy, tired, agitated, or in pain. A brief session helps to make the program more manageable.

2. Communicate clearly and use simple language. Patients have experienced cognitive impairments, so simplifying concepts is better. At times, the patient may appear disengaged or fall asleep, so it is fine to focus more on caregivers in Session 1. There is ample opportunity to teach and re-teach skills in future sessions.

3. Build a strong therapeutic alliance with the dyad. Many dyads are receptive to support during hospitalization; however, it can be hard to maintain participation after discharge. Strong rapport helps with engagement and retention.

4. The ICU is a fast-paced unit, and many different providers are involved in the patient's care. Work closely with the ICU team to coordinate care in a way that works best for that unit. Check in with bedside nurses to determine optimal timing for the session and provide them with updates after the session. If social work is involved, communicate the plan and updates with them as well. Another option is to write a brief note in the patient's electronic medical record.

5. Be friendly and assertive. Psychosocial care is rarely embedded in these settings, so create time and space for this service and educate dyads and staff. Psychoeducation on the mind–body connection and interdisciplinary care can help promote buy-in.

6. Flexibility is key. Be familiar with and respectful of the acuity of the medical care. When emergency situations occur, adapt the session as needed. In addition, adapt the material however you see fit. Although we provide scripts throughout the session, they are only examples. It is most important to be authentic to your clinical style. This session is meant to be flexible, as long as you deliver the skills.

Logistics for Delivery

Ideally, the session is delivered at the bedside with both dyad members present. However, if caregivers cannot come to the unit for the session, they can join virtually (over a live video platform, such as Zoom). If they do not have access to live video, they can join by phone. Sometimes patients are discharged shortly after program enrollment and before Session 1. In these instances, you can conduct the session over live video with both dyad members. If possible, meet with them and schedule the appointment prior to their discharge. Dyads have a lot to manage after discharge, so meeting them in person during hospitalization helps build rapport. Remember to confirm that they can access the live video platform or have support to access it.

Assessment and Chart Review

Prior to each session, ensure that each dyad member completes the validated measures of depression and anxiety (Hospital Anxiety and Depression Scale [HADS]) and posttraumatic stress (Posttraumatic Stress Disorder Checklist for DSM-5 [PCL-5]). You can send the measures over email prior to each session or have the dyad complete them at the beginning of each session. Regular assessment of symptoms allows you to track progress and tailor the skills to help address specific symptoms.

The measures are included at the beginning of each session. The items of these measures correspond to symptoms. Reviewing them helps you to tailor the content to address the dyad's needs. For example, on the HADS, if they endorse more anxiety symptoms such as feeling "tense or wound up," then explain how Deep Breathing can help reduce physiological arousal. You can also spend more time on the skills that are most relevant to their current distress because this will facilitate home practice. You can also use the exact symptoms they endorse as examples when explaining the skills.

In addition to reviewing assessments, review the patient's medical record to understand their reason for admission, medical history, and relevant psychosocial background. However, do not offer any medical information to dyads because this is outside the scope of this program. The medical team will update them as they see fit. If dyads ask about plans for medical care, explain your role and encourage them to ask their team about any medical-related questions.

Session 1

The rest of this chapter aligns with Session 1 in the Workbook. Refer the dyad to page 5 in their Workbook. By searching for this book's title on the Oxford Academic platform at academic.oup.com, the dyad will have access to explainer videos pertaining to each skill they will learn in Recovering Together. They can reference these videos to learn new skills and to review skills learned in previous sessions. They will also have access to audio recordings, which will help them practice skills they learn.

The web resources accompanying Session 1 are:

- Deep Breathing Explainer Video
- Deep Breathing Exercise Audio
- Diaphragmatic Breathing Audio
- Mindfulness Meditation Instructions Audio
- Mindfulness Meditation Practice Audio
- Mountain Meditation Audio
- Mindfulness Meditation 2 Audio

In the Workbook, the content is presented as:

- What It Is
- How It Helps
- When to Use It
- How to Use It

These sections can be delivered in any order based on your clinical judgment. Reinforce anything that you see as positive in the patient and caregiver. We want them to feel better about themselves during the recovery process. Although we present scripts below, these are provided as examples. We encourage you to adapt them to fit your style and the dyad's needs.

Introductions and Rapport-Building

Begin by introducing yourself and your role. Explain the value of the Recovering Together program. Make sure each member of the dyad understands why this program will help them as individuals and as a unit.

Hi, [NAMES], I'm [NAME]. I will be your clinician for the Recovering Together program. I'm looking forward to working with you both over the next 6 weeks. It is great that you are interested in this program because it has been shown to reduce distress and improve recovery. The goal of this program is to teach skills that will help you manage the stress that comes along with being in the hospital and adjusting to life after. The fact that you are participating together is so valuable because it will help you learn how to cope as individuals and together. Research shows that using positive coping skills helps improve emotional functioning for each of you individually, and together. Your emotional recovery is interrelated. When one of you does better, both of you do better. So, let's get started. First, I'll provide an overview of the program and then we'll jump into the agenda for Session 1.

Overview and Rationale of Program

Provide an overview of the program (structure and materials). Suggest that the dyad review this information on pages 2–3 in the Workbook. Orient them to the Workbook for weekly assessment and home practice. Answer any questions they have about the program.

You will both participate in six 30- to 45-minute weekly sessions. The first two sessions will occur in person (unless you are discharged before then). The latter four (or more) will occur over Zoom. The program is customized. After the first two sessions, we will choose together four out of five sessions. This program is skills-based, meaning that we will learn and practice skills that will help optimize your recovery and adjustment. It involves your active participation. In each session we'll review prior skills, discuss new skills, practice them together, and make a plan for the week. Between sessions, you will have access to videos and recordings that further explain the skills and offer opportunities to practice. These can be accessed by searching for this book's title on the Oxford Academic plat-form at academic.oup.com.

Practicing between sessions will help you get the most out of this pro-gram. It will also help you feel that you are actively participating in your recovery. The program skills are meant to be practiced anywhere, any-time, and for as little as a couple of minutes. We will figure out together how to help you incorporate the program skills smoothly into your busy lives. Most importantly, we want this to be helpful for your journey. Ask questions, give feedback, and let me know which skills are most helpful. We can tailor the program accordingly.

What questions do you have for me?

Agenda

Orient the dyad to Session 1 in their Workbooks. Explain that there are pictures (icons) to represent the skills and each week new skills will be added. Explain that they are building a skillset and by the end of the program, they will have many skills to choose from to enhance recovery and life in general.

Open your Workbooks to Session 1 (page 5). As you can see, there are pictures to represent the skills of the session. Each week, you will learn skills that will build on each other. The prior session's skills and the new skills will be displayed at the start of each session. By the end, you will have developed a skillset, allowing you to choose which skills to use. Using these skills in everyday life will help improve your recovery and living in general.

Review the agenda for the session. Agenda-setting helps set expecta-tions for the session. It allows you to respectfully move on to new topics within the session timeframe.

If you turn to page 8, you will see the agenda for today. We will discuss your experience so far and common challenges for patients and caregivers. Then, we will discuss and practice skills including Deep Breathing, Mindful Stoplight, Staying in the 24-Hour Block, and Mindfulness Meditation. Finally, we will discuss ways to practice these skills over the next week.

Ask the dyad about their hospitalization and current concerns and challenges. Normalize and validate their experiences. Provide psychoeducation about common individual and shared experiences (see page 9 of the Workbook). Make sure they understand that stress is interdependent (which is why their mutual participation is important). Explain that the goal of the Recovering Together treatment program is to optimize emotional function as individuals and together because this will help physical function.

How has your experience been thus far?

If they need prompting, encourage them to review the Workbook and provide examples.

There are many factors that impact the hospital stay and adjustment. Take a look at the information displayed on page 9 in your Workbooks and the picture below. What jumps out at you as relevant to your experience as individuals and as a unit?

Encourage both dyad members to share their experiences. If one tends to be more talkative, then ask the other member about their perspective. When possible, give opportunities for both dyad members to share their experience and encourage active listening to one another. Make sure that the program is tailored for both patients and caregivers and encourage their interactions and communications. Often caregivers are reluctant to share their own distress because of fear of upsetting the patient. Normalize this and reinforce honesty and support.

[PATIENT], what has your experience been like? [CAREGIVER], what about for you?

After they have each shared, move on to the skills for this first session.

We are now going to discuss the session skills, which will serve as a foundation for the later sessions.

Deep Breathing

Introduce Deep Breathing and explain how it helps. Emphasize that breathing from the belly (diaphragm) rather than from the chest signals to our body (parasympathetic system) to move into the relaxation state. This is important during times of stress.

> *When we experience stress, our breathing automatically becomes shallow and rapid. This type of breathing makes us anxious and fearful. If we take a few deep, slow breaths from our belly, we can reboot our system and can start feeling relaxed and calm. Is this something you have done?*

Be sure to practice Deep Breathing *experientially*. Guide them through a practice or use the Deep Breathing Exercise Audio Recording (which can be accessed by searching for this book's title on the Oxford Academic platform at academic.oup.com). To enhance the exercise, ask them to notice how they are feeling before and after the exercise (0 to 10 scale of distress). So before practicing, ask the dyad how they are feeling right now using the term "emotional distress" or any term they used to describe their experience (e.g., "stress," "anxiety").

> *On a scale of 1 to 10, how much emotional distress [anxiety, stress] are you experiencing right now?*

> *Let's use the recording right now and practice together.*

After the exercise, ask the dyad the same question:

> *Now, on a scale of 1 to 10, how much emotional distress [anxiety, stress] are you experiencing right now?*

Validate their responses and offer suggestions to improve the experience. For example, if they note that there are distractions (e.g., sounds, thoughts), suggest that they count during each inhale and exhale or notice how their belly expands. Explain that the more they practice, the more it will help. Discuss when they can use Deep Breathing in daily life. Link the opportunity to practice Deep Breathing with items that they endorse on the HADS anxiety scale or PCL-5.

Mindful Stoplight

Ask the dyad about their understanding of mindfulness.

We're going to talk about our next skill, which is mindfulness. Have you heard of mindfulness before?

Have you ever used mindfulness? In what ways? How was that?

Correct or build on their definition of mindfulness. Explain that being nonjudgmental and curious is important for mindfulness. Ensure that the dyad understands the benefits of it.

Mindfulness means tuning in to the present moment. Our minds tend to focus on the past and the future, which is not always helpful. Often, we are not even aware of this—we are on autopilot. In times of stress our minds are good about coming up with the worst-case scenarios. These scenarios create anxiety, fear, and worries. These worst-case scenarios most often don't come true, and they negatively impact recovery. What do you think about this?

Mindfulness allows us to take control over our minds and bring them back to the present moment. Mindfulness grounds us in the present. A common misconception is that mindfulness means having a clear mind with no thoughts. This is not true. However, mindfulness allows us to notice, without judgment, what is happening in our body, mind, and the environment. Embracing a nonjudgmental and curious attitude is important. This helps create space from our thoughts and feelings, which then provides us with more time to decide how to move forward. It is interesting what our minds can come up with, the stories they can create!

Mindfulness is very helpful in situations of high stress like the Neuro-ICU. Being aware and accepting our experiences helps reduce stress, which improves our ability to make decisions and communicate with our loved ones and the team. Mindfulness can seem abstract, so let's practice together. Turn to page 10 in your Workbooks.

Introduce the Mindful Stoplight metaphor to explain the three aspects of mindfulness. Be consistent with the language in the Workbook and keep it simple.

For this program, we are going to talk about mindfulness with the image of a stoplight. This picture will help you remember the term *mindfulness and how to practice it. As you can see, **Observe** is the red light: Stop. This is a reminder to pause and notice, without words, and with curiosity toward your experiences. These can be internal (thoughts, feelings, body sensations) or external (your room). **Describe** is the yellow light: Continue to pause. Once you've noticed what's going on, be intentional about describing experiences without judgment. Be curious and label experiences with fact (without judgment) to create a healthy separation from them. For example, we can practice labeling our thoughts: "I'm having the thought that I won't recover" or "I'm having the thought that my partner won't recover." Finally, **Act with Awareness** is the green light: Go. Once we have observed and described our experiences, we can now proceed forward and engage with our experiences in a way that is consistent with our values and long-term goals.*

If needed, provide an example (from the Workbook or another one). Encourage each dyad member to practice (written or verbally) with their own example. Make sure they both participate (if the patient is awake and able to engage). Normalize the experience.

Now, let's practice together. Turn to page 12 in your Workbooks. Can you each [write down or share] your own example? What are you observing (red light)? Can you describe it (yellow light)? How will you proceed (green light)?

Reflect on this practice. Ask them how they feel at the end of the exercise. Ideally, they had a good experience and realize that by tuning in to their experiences they can better manage them. The goal is that they understand and buy into the value of mindfulness. You do not want them to leave feeling like mindfulness is still an abstract idea, but rather something they can incorporate into everyday life.

Staying in the 24-Hour Block

Introduce the skill of Staying in the 24-Hour Block. Dyads often feel overwhelmed about what might happen during and after hospitalization. Things constantly change in the ICU, so focusing on one day at a time is essential. Explain that this can apply to the day or even to the next hour, minute, second, or moment, and that mindfulness helps us stay in these time periods.

This next skill (Staying in the 24-Hour Block) is particularly helpful for your time in the hospital and after you leave. Many dyads feel overwhelmed with the uncertainty of the situation or fear about the future. Your minds are at work creating worst-case scenarios. Right now, you might be experiencing heightened worry as you think about the future and navigate changes. This skill helps you stay in the present, prioritize what is important now, help manage emotions, and learn how to best support each other. Although the skill is called Staying in the 24-Hour Block, you can use this flexibly. There may be times when you can only focus on staying within the next hour, the next 10 minutes, or even the next moment. The goal is to do what you can to shift away from unhelpful thoughts about the future or past. You can use this skill any time you find yourself feeling overwhelmed or stuck in thoughts about the future or past.

Then, use the Mindful Stoplight (page 13 in the Workbook) as an example of how to use this skill.

You might observe a thought like "I notice I am thinking far into the future." The next step would be describing it. You might label it as "worry about the future," and tell yourself that it is normal to have that thought. Then you can act with awareness. You may consider practicing Deep Breathing or using the Recovering Together audio recordings, which can be accessed by searching for this book's title on the Oxford Academic platform at academic.oup.com. Reducing physical arousal will help you figure out what you can do today to best prepare for the future.

Mindfulness Meditation

Explain that meditation is mindfulness for a longer amount of time. If time allows, deliver this exercise in the hospital room. You can use your own meditation or play the Mindfulness Meditation Practice Audio Recordings, which can be accessed by searching for this book's title on the Oxford Academic platform at academic.oup.com. Emphasize that they can practice mindfulness in a busy hospital (or anywhere) together. Encourage them to listen to the guided practice.

Mindfulness Meditation is mindfulness for a longer amount of time. This skill can help you use mindfulness to regulate your emotions and stay within the 24-hour block. This skill is most helpful with regular practice. You can access the Mindfulness Meditation Practice Audio Recordings by searching for this book's title on the Oxford Academic platform at academic.oup.com. You can practice mindfulness alone or together anywhere, such as bedside, rehab, or home.

Session 1 Summary

At the end of session, thank dyad members for their participation. Instill confidence in their ability to apply what they've learned. Orient them to the Session 1 summary and the table of skills in the Workbook. Explain that a table of the skills is presented at the end of each session for quick review. Ask about their reactions to the skills and which may be most useful. Explain that different skills work for different people, so our goal is to figure out which work best for them.

Thank you both for your participation today. I am confident that you will master these skills and find them useful during this time and beyond. On pages 14–15 in your Workbooks, there is an overview of the session and the skills we practiced today. At the end of each session, there will be a table of new skills so you can quickly reference it during the week. So far, which skills do you like the best? Which ones will be most useful over the next week?

After reviewing the skills, encourage the patient and caregiver to access videos and recordings that will help them practice by searching for this book's title on the Oxford Academic platform at academic.oup.com. Make sure at least one dyad member can access the website on their phone, tablet, or computer.

Prescription for Recovery (Home Practice)

Explain the weekly Prescription for Recovery. Encourage the dyad to practice the skills over the next week to figure out which work for them. Explain that this will help you tailor the program to best meet their needs. Ask when they might practice skills using the support materials (which they can access by searching for this book's title on the Oxford Academic platform at academic.oup.com).

At the end of each session, you will see the Prescription for Recovery. We have learned that practice is necessary to make skills a part of everyday life, and I'm here to support you to build those skills. In the Prescription for Recovery sections, you can take notes about skills to practice, goals for your practice for skills, and any questions that come up between sessions. For today's session, you may take notes on how you can use Deep Breathing, Mindful Stoplight, Staying in the 24-Hour Block, or Mindfulness Meditation. Throughout the week, you can take notes on how you've practiced individually and together. And make sure to write anything down that you'd like to review in the next session. Do you have ideas of how you can apply the skills over the next week?

Work with the patient and caregiver to commit to practice at least one skill over the next week and make a plan to keep each other accountable with practice, when appropriate. Some dyads like to practice together, while others want to practice on their own. Remind them that practice is flexible, and they can do it anywhere and at any time. Remind them about the website to facilitate practice.

And remember that the website can help you practice. We created recordings that you can listen to during your hospital stay and after; these recordings can be accessed by searching for this book's title on the Oxford Academic platform at academic.oup.com. It might be difficult, but if you can practice mindfulness here in the hospital, you can practice anywhere.

Schedule Next Session

Make sure that you schedule Session 2. Session 2 can occur in the hospital or virtually (depending on whether the patient is discharged). Depending on their discharge plans and preference, Session 2 can occur any time after completion of this session (e.g., next day). You can share your professional contact information (email, phone) if you are comfortable doing so.

Our sessions will be weekly. However, we can schedule Session 2 earlier if you prefer to meet in person. Which do you prefer? When works for you both? [If next week], do you have access to Zoom [or another virtual platform]?

Answer their questions and remind them that they will receive an email to complete the measures prior to the next session. End the session in a way that helps instill hope.

Do you have any final questions? Feel free to email or call me if anything changes or you need anything. Also, before the next session, you will receive an email from me to complete the same measures prior to the next session. This helps me understand how you are each doing and tailor the program accordingly.

It was wonderful to meet you both! I look forward to working together and seeing your progress. I know that you'll find this program helpful, especially during this transition time. I'll see you on [DATE] at [TIME], and please reach out at any point.

CHAPTER 2

Session 2: Coping with Uncertainty

(Corresponds to Session 2 of the Workbook)

Materials

- Clinician Guide and Workbooks
- Pens

Outline of Session 2

Session 2 Goals

Preparing for Session 2
- Recommendations for Clinicians
- Logistics for Delivery
- Assessment (administer and/or review measures of depression, anxiety, and posttraumatic stress for each dyad member)

Session 2

Agenda

Check In and Review Session 1 and Prescription for Recovery (Home Practice)

Skills (Teach and Practice)
- Dialectics: Seeing Multiple Sides
- Hands as Worries

Session 2 Summary

Prescription for Recovery (Home Practice)

Schedule Next Session

1. Build rapport with the dyad. Dyads are most likely to drop out after Session 2 (often taking place in the hospital) and before Session 3 (at a rehabilitation center or home) given the challenges of this transition. A strong therapeutic alliance helps keep them engaged in the program.
2. Ensure that dyad members understand the importance of home practice. Take time to review Session 1 skills and problem-solve ways that they can practice in the hospital and after discharge. Encourage them to practice individually and together.
3. Teach skills in a way that the dyad can understand. Make the skills, especially Dialectics, concrete by sharing examples. Encourage the patient and caregiver to come up their own examples. Dialectics is foundational to this program, so it is important that they understand how it applies to everyday life and ways to use it.

Preparing for Session 2

Recommendations for Clinicians

Consistent with Session 1, it is important to build rapport with the dyad. Session 2 has fewer skills and allows for time to review Session 1 and discuss strategies for home practice. Patients may have been less engaged in Session 1, so the review of Session 1 skills is important. It can be difficult to practice skills in the hospital, so practice with the dyad in session. For example, if you notice anxiety, consider practicing Deep Breathing with them; if you notice waning attention, lead them through a brief mindfulness exercise. Further, many patients will be experiencing cognitive impairments or will be in pain or fatigued. Explain skills clearly and as simply as possible. If you notice limitations in thinking or speech, go slow and check in often with the dyad. Session 2 is either delivered in the hospital or after discharge (see "Logistics for Delivery" below). If they are discharged (at a rehabilitation center or home), when you introduce skills, discuss what the dyad noticed in the hospital and what they notice now. Discuss ways that they can create time and space to practice (privacy, quiet space, reliable internet) across settings.

As mentioned in Session 1, adapt the material however you see fit. Although we provide scripts throughout the session, they are provided as examples. It is most important to be authentic to your clinical style. This session is meant to be flexible, as long as you deliver the program skills.

Logistics for Delivery

If the patient is still in the hospital, Session 2 is delivered at the bedside, ideally with both dyad members present. If caregivers cannot come to the unit for the session, they can join virtually (over a live video platform, such as Zoom). If they do not have access to live video, they can join by phone. If the patient has been discharged, conduct the session over live video with both dyad members.

Assessment

Prior to the session, review each dyad member's responses to the validated measures of depression and anxiety (Hospital Anxiety and Depression Scale [HADS]) and posttraumatic stress (Posttraumatic Stress Disorder Checklist for DSM-5 [PCL-5]) (see the introductory chapter for details on assessments). You can send the measures over email prior to each session or have the dyad complete them at the beginning of each session. Regular assessment of symptoms allows you to track progress and tailor the skills to help address specific symptoms.

The measures are also included on pages 18–19 of the Workbook. The items of these measures correspond to symptoms. Reviewing them helps you tailor the content to address the dyad's needs. For example, on the HADS, if they endorse more anxiety symptoms such as feeling "tense or wound up," then explain how Deep Breathing can help reduce physiological arousal. You can also spend more time on the skills that are most relevant to their current distress because this will facilitate home practice. You can also use the exact symptoms they endorse as examples when explaining the skills.

Session 2

The rest of this chapter aligns with Session 2 in the workbook. Refer the dyad to page 17 in their Workbook. By searching for this book's title on the Oxford Academic platform at academic.oup.com, the dyad will have access to explainer videos pertaining to each skill they will learn in Recovering Together. They can reference these videos to learn new skills and to review skills learned in previous sessions. They will also have access to audio recordings, which will help them practice the skills they learn in Recovering Together.

The web resources accompanying Session 2 are:

- Dialectics Explainer Video
- Hands as Worries Audio

In the Workbook, the content is presented as:

- What It Is
- How It Helps
- When to Use It
- How to Use It

These sections can be delivered in any order based on your clinical judgment. Although we present scripts throughout this Clinician Guide, these are provided as examples. We encourage you to adapt them to fit your style and the dyad's needs.

Agenda

Orient the dyad to Session 2 in their workbooks. Remind them that the pictures represent the skills and new ones are added each week. Encourage them to practice and identify the ones that are most helpful.

Open your workbooks to Session 2 (page 17). As a reminder, the pictures represent the skills from the prior and current sessions. These skills build on each other, and I encourage you to try them all and see which work best for you.

Review the agenda with the dyad before checking in on the last session, skills practice, and any significant emotional distress or medical complications.

If you turn to page 20, you will see the agenda for today. We will review the materials discussed last week and then discuss new skills. Today, we will be learning about Dialectics and practicing the Hands as Worries skill.

Check In and Review Session 1 and Prescription for Recovery (Home Practice)

Check in with the dyad to see how they are doing. Often things have changed for them. They may have been moved to a different floor, may have been discharged to rehab or home, or may have received disappointing news (e.g., new diagnosis). Allowing space for dyads to catch you up to speed is helpful and will enhance their engagement. Be sure you have reviewed their medical chart before this session (if available).

Thank you for being here today. How are you each doing today? How have things changed since last week?

Briefly review Session 1 skills. Explain the value of home practice.

In our last session, we discussed the skills of Deep Breathing, Mindful Stoplight, Staying in the 24-Hour Block, and Mindfulness Meditation. We discussed what they are, how they are helpful, and when they can be used. It is important to try them outside of session. You can think of it as a little experiment to figure out which skills work for you. Practicing them regularly (not only when you are stressed) helps them become second nature. The more you practice, the easier these skills will part of your "toolkit" that you can use when you are feeling stressed.

Ask the dyad if they were able to practice the skills. Discuss ways that they practiced.

What do you both think of these skills? Were you able to practice any of the skills? How did that go?

If the dyad practiced any skills, validate their practice. Explore how they practiced and which skills they used. Ask whether they noticed any changes after using the skills.

That's amazing! Which skills did you practice? When did you use them? Did you practice individually or together? Did you notice any change after?

If the dyad did not practice, validate the challenges of practicing. Reiterate the value of practice.

It can be hard to practice with everything going on (especially in the ICU). Practicing the skills helps you learn how they can be applied into your daily lives. Often, different skills work for different people, so practicing also helps us figure out which are most helpful to you as individuals and as a unit. Let's problem-solve together how to make it part of your routine.

Help the patient and caregiver problem-solve their reported barriers. Use the "Be Strategic" section (Workbook page 20) to create a plan to practice. Reinforce the plan at the end of the session. Review the tips for and value of practicing together.

What will help you practice? When can you practice? Where can you do it?

Practicing the skills together is a valuable way to hold each other accountable. You can remind each other and integrate the skills into a routine (such as listening to a meditation at night). What are some ways that you can practice together or help remind each other?

Skills (Teach and Practice)

Dialectics: Seeing Multiple Sides

Introduce Dialectics as a foundational skill for the program. This concept can be difficult to understand, so try to keep the explanation clear and simple. Try using different terms to describe it, such as contradictions, multiple truths, "both sides of the coin," "feeling it all," or pieces of a puzzle. If the dyad understands the concept, there's no need to use different terms. If they do not, then try describing it in other ways.

However, do not overwhelm them. It is better to practice and learn it with examples. Offer examples and encourage the patient and caregiver to come up with their own.

> *The first skill for today is called Dialectics. Have you heard the word Dialectics before? Dialectics is a word that means contradictions. In other words, multiple things (even if they seem conflicting) can be true at the same time. For example, many patients report feeling angry that this event happened AND grateful that they are alive. Caregivers often say that they want to express their stress to their loved one AND do not want to burden them. Have you noticed any thoughts or feelings that seem to be at odds with each other?*

If dyad members have trouble understanding, try explaining in different ways. For example, ask what would happen if we only focused on one side (e.g., if we were only ever happy, or only sad). Discuss how both need to exist. Below are a few additional ways to explain it.

> *Sometimes it is helpful to think about what life would be like if only one side exists. For example, what if we were only ever happy? Or only ever sad? We probably would not even know the other emotion. And as we all know, we all experience many emotions.*

> *Sometimes the yin-yang symbol is used to represent Dialectics. This is because it shows that light and dark coexist. We need to acknowledge the good and bad. We have both good and bad experiences, emotions, and thoughts. All of them can coexist, and that is part of what makes life interesting and rewarding.*

Explain the value of Dialectics (example below). If the dyad offered examples, then use those to explain the importance of seeing and accepting multiple perspectives or experiences. If needed, normalize that Dialectics or contradictory thoughts can be confusing. Explain how accepting contradictory thoughts can help us be more flexible in our thinking.

> *Dialectics helps us get out from having to choose the "right" side or one single "truth" in our way of viewing things. Identifying Dialectics allows us to accept that there can be multiple truths and can help us see the bigger picture. It gives us more flexibility in how we view ourselves and allows us to accept our experiences and our partners.*

Explain how the patient and caregiver can practice Dialectics. Practice replacing "but" with "and" in session together.

So how can we practice Dialectics? It is actually very simple! Often when we are describing conflicting thoughts or emotions, we use the word "but." For example, someone might say, "I understand that you are upset, but I did not mean to hurt you." In this instance, the "but" negates the first part of the sentence. It sounds like they are discounting the other person's experience. To make room for all perspectives, a trick is to replace the word "but" with "and." In this example, it would become "I understand that you are upset AND I did not mean to hurt you." Changing "but" to "and" allows for both experiences to be true. What are your reactions? Can you think of any examples?

Discuss when the dyad can practice Dialectics. Explain that it may feel odd at first AND it will become more natural as they practice. Encourage them to identify times that Dialectics can be helpful.

Dialectics is useful when you're having multiple emotions or thoughts that seem like they're at odds with one another. It might feel strange AND the more you do it, the more natural it will feel. Can you think of a time when Dialectics would be helpful?

Orient the dyad to the "Dialectics Are Like a Puzzle" section on page 23 in the Workbook. Read that section verbatim to introduce the puzzle metaphor. Ask the patient and caregiver to observe what thoughts and emotions are coming up.

Now, turn to page 23 in your Workbooks. As you can see, there is an image of a puzzle. Dialectics are like a puzzle. Each puzzle piece represents a different thought or emotion. When you first open the box, it can be overwhelming. We might want to avoid doing the puzzle. With time, we learn to accept the different pieces. Part of our work together is recognizing and creating space from each puzzle piece (or difficult thought or emotion) so that we can see the bigger picture. I encourage you to help each other do that so you can focus on what is important or the bigger picture.

Ask the dyad to identify their "puzzle pieces" (thoughts and emotions during the hospital stay or at the current time). Have them describe their puzzle pieces to each other using "and." If they are having trouble, then offer an example from the workbook. Emphasize AND with your voice (volume, tone) to help the dyad notice Dialectics.

What are some thoughts or emotions that are coming up for each of you? Can you describe them using the word "and"?

Validate their practice and offer suggestions if they are having trouble. Ask the dyad for their preferred term for Dialectics and then use that throughout the program. Encourage them to review the Dialectics Explainer Video by searching for this book's title on the Oxford Academic platform at academic.oup.com.

Hands as Worries

Introduce the Hands as Worries skill. Explain that when we are worried, we can be preoccupied about the future. As a result, we may isolate from others or appear preoccupied. Ask them each to identify a worry.

When we get preoccupied about the future, we sometimes feel distant from others. It is normal to worry AND sometimes when we get stuck on worries it can be difficult to separate from worrying thoughts. What is the most difficult worry for each of you right now?

Explain why this skill is helpful. Discuss how it promotes acceptance. Explain what acceptance means in this context and how it helps us to be more present in our lives.

This skill helps promote acceptance. Worries are a part of life and will come and go. Accepting worries does not mean that we like them or approve them; it simply means not avoiding or pushing away what has already happened. This is important because when we become all-consumed by worries, then we are missing out on time with our loved ones or doing things we enjoy. This skill allows us to notice and create space from worries. As a result, we can be more present so we can live our lives more fully, even with the worries.

Discuss when to use this skill.

You can use this skill when you observe that you are distracted or consumed with worry or anxiety. This is a way of acting with awareness—when you practice Hands as Worries, you are allowing your worry to exist while moving forward with your life and trying to see the bigger picture.

Lead them through the exercise on page 24 of the Workbook. Take a light-hearted approach and encourage the dyad to laugh and joke with one another.

Let's try this exercise together so you learn how to use it. [Read the script verbatim from the workbook on page 24].

Ask the dyad for their impressions.

How was that exercise for each of you? When might this skill be useful?

Explain how Mindful Stoplight skills (observe, describe) can help us notice where our hands are in different moments. Discuss how the dyad can use this skill to gently remind themselves or each other to "hold their worries lightly."

It is useful to think about how this skill builds on other ones. Noticing where our hands are in the first place requires a level of curious awareness that is fostered by mindfulness. Our observing skills help us notice when we are worrying in the first place. You can also help each other notice. Many dyads adopt the phrase: "Where are my hands right now?" This can be applied to yourself or to each other. In this way, you can help each other navigate fears and worries throughout recovery.

Encourage the dyad to review the Hands as Worries Audio Recording for practice by searching for this book's title on the Oxford Academic platform at academic.oup.com).

Session 2 Summary

Orient the patient and caregiver to the summary and table of skills at the end of Session 2 in the Workbook. Briefly review the session content and skills.

On page 25 in your Workbooks, there is a summary of our session. This table is a great way to quickly reference skills. Today, we learned the benefits of mindfulness and how you can practice individually and together. We also discussed new skills to navigate uncertainty and complex experiences. Dialectics helps us accept and be curious about seemingly opposing thoughts and feelings. It can be as simple as replacing a "but" with an "and." The Hands as Worries skill can help you be more flexible during times of stress. It can be helpful to practice individually and together.

Ask the dyad which skill(s) they want to practice over the next week. Explore how they might build on the skills they learned in the prior session.

So far, which skills do you like the best? Which ones will be most useful over the next week?

Prescription for Recovery (Home Practice)

Remind the dyad about the weekly Prescription for Recovery section. Ask for specific times that they will plan to use the skills.

As we go along, the Prescription for Recovery is a helpful reminder to practice the skills, including those from prior sessions (Deep Breathing, Mindful Stoplight, Staying in the 24-Hour Block, and Mindfulness Meditation) and the new ones from today (Dialectics and Hands as Worries). You can take notes about skills to practice, goals for your practice for skills, and any questions that come up between sessions. Do you have ideas of how you can apply the skills over the next week?

When appropriate, encourage the patient and caregiver to keep each other accountable with practice. Remind them that practice is flexible, and they can do it anywhere and at any time.

It can be helpful to plan times to practice together (or individually). That way, you can help hold each other accountable. Remember, you can practice the skills anytime and anywhere—the goal is to make them a part of everyday life.

Remind the dyad to practice the skills using the materials they can access by searching for this book's title on the Oxford Academic platform at academic.oup.com.

Remember that the website can facilitate practice. We created recordings that can be accessed by searching for this book's title on the Oxford Academic platform at academic.oup.com.

Schedule Next Session

Because this program is modular, you will select the rest of the sessions with the dyad. Together you can choose four of the possible five sessions. Before ending Session 2, make sure to ask the dyad for their preferences for their next sessions (see the "Your Sessions" chart on page 3 in the Workbook).

Now that we have completed Sessions 1 and 2, we will choose the rest of the sessions together. Go to page 3 in your Workbooks to review a list of possible sessions. We will do four of the five listed. Are there any that stand out as particularly useful or not useful?

If they are not sure, then encourage them to do Session 3 because it helps set the foundation for other sessions. If they identify one session that is less relevant to them, then skip that one and do the rest in the order provided.

For next week, we can continue with Session 3 (Adjusting to Life After an Acute Neurological Illness [ANI]) or do any of the others. If you think Session 3 would be helpful, I recommend that we do that one next. What do you both think?

Remind the dyad that the rest of the sessions will occur virtually. If needed, check in that the dyad knows how to navigate Zoom. Schedule the session for next week.

The rest of our sessions will be remote (over Zoom). Do you have Zoom? Do you have any questions about it?

When works for you both next week?

End the session by thanking the dyad for their participation. Answer their questions and remind them that they will receive an email to complete the measures prior to the next session.

Thank you for your participation today! Do you have any final questions? Feel free to email or call me if anything changes or you need anything. Also, before the next session, you will receive an email from me to complete the same measures prior to the next session. This helps me understand how you are each doing and tailor the program accordingly. I'll see you on [DATE] and [TIME], and please reach out at any point.

CHAPTER 3

Session 3: Adjusting to Life After an Acute Neurological Illness (ANI)

(Corresponds to Session 3 of the Workbook)

Materials

- Clinician Guide and Workbooks
- Pens

Outline of Session 3

Session 3 Goals

Preparing for Session 3

- Recommendations for Clinicians
- Logistics for Delivery
- Assessment (administer and/or review measures of depression, anxiety, and posttraumatic stress for each dyad member)

Session 3

Agenda

Check In and Review Prior Session and Prescription for Recovery (Home Practice)

Skills (Teach and Practice)

- Understanding Your and Your Partner's Stressors
- Identifying the Distress Spiral
- Challenging Unhelpful Thoughts After ANI

Session 3 Summary

Prescription for Recovery (Home Practice)

Schedule Next Session

1. Continue to build rapport with the dyad. Dyads are most likely to drop out after Session 2 (often taking place in the hospital) and before Session 3 (at a rehabilitation center or home) given the challenges of this transition. A strong therapeutic alliance helps keep them engaged in the program.

2. Allow for flexibility with scheduling. Because Session 3 is often scheduled when dyads are still in the hospital and are unclear about their schedules when they transition to rehab or home, they may cancel or fail to show up at the third session. Be flexible and accommodate their schedules. Consider a check in between Sessions 2 and 3 to confirm or adjust the date/time for Session 3.

3. Continue reinforcing the importance of home practice. Take time to review Session 2 skills and problem-solve ways that the patient and caregiver can practice after discharge. Many of their "practice cues" are going to change after discharge. Help them develop new habits around home practice. Encourage them to practice individually and together.

4. Teach skills by applying them to the individual challenges of each dyad. Ensure that dyads understand the skills of Sessions 1 and 2. These skills are core skills and will continue to be used in Session 3 and across all sessions. Focus on experiential learning and encourage the dyad to come up with their own examples.

Preparing for Session 3

Recommendations for Clinicians

Consistent with Sessions 1 and 2, it is important to continue building rapport with the dyad. This session is also typically the first session after discharge. Dyads might have looked forward to discharge, which symbolizes that the patient is well enough to go to rehab or home. However, once home, dyads can experience increased anxiety because they have lost the safety of on-call medical care. The caregiver now faces the reality of being 100% in charge of the care, and they may not have time off from work or additional support. It is important to understand the individual situation of each dyad. It is also important to understand where they are in the physical recovery journey—sometimes dyads have made the most recovery in the hospital, other times recovery will continue at home for many more months.

Session 3 gives you an opportunity to learn about these details through the Distress Spiral—understanding negative thoughts, unpleasant emotions, and unhelpful behaviors. Home practice is also often impacted by the move to rehab or home. It is important to discuss this transition with the dyad and help them set up new habits for home practice. As in every session, pay attention to the patient–caregiver interactions and focus on preserving or enhancing their relationship. Approaching the recovery as a team is key. By this session, typically the patient can be more engaged and able to engage with higher-level skills. Nonetheless, it is still important to explain skills clearly and ensure that the dyad understands them. Make sure that the caregiver gets as much space as the patient—often caregivers tend to feel less worthy of attention and care since they did not experience the acute neurological illness (ANI).

As mentioned in prior sessions, adapt the material however you see fit. Although we provide scripts throughout the session, they are provided as examples. It is most important to be authentic to your clinical style. This session is meant to be flexible, as long as you deliver the program skills.

Logistics for Delivery

This may be the first session that is delivered via Zoom. The patient and caregiver may or may not be together.

Assessment

Prior to the session, review each dyad member's responses to the validated measures of depression and anxiety (Hospital Anxiety and Depression Scale [HADS]) and posttraumatic stress (Posttraumatic Stress Disorder Checklist for DSM-5 [PCL-5]) (see Introduction for details on assessments). You can send the measures over email prior to each session or have the dyad complete them at the beginning of each session. Regular assessment of symptoms allows you to track progress and tailor the skills to help address specific symptoms.

The measures are also included on pages 28–29 of the Workbook. The items of these measures correspond to symptoms. Reviewing them informs how to tailor the content to address the dyad's needs. For example, on the HADS, if they endorse more anxiety symptoms such as feeling "tense or wound up," then explain how Deep Breathing can help reduce physiological arousal. You can also spend more time on skills that are most relevant to their current distress because this will facilitate home practice. You can also the exact symptoms they endorse as examples when explaining skills. Their responses on the HADS and PCL-5 can also be helpful in this session in case the dyad has trouble identifying negative thoughts, unpleasant emotions, and unhelpful behaviors.

Session 3

The rest of this chapter aligns with Session 3 in the workbook. Refer the dyad to page 27 in their Workbook. By searching for this book's title on the Oxford Academic platform at academic.oup.com, the dyad will have access to explainer videos pertaining to each skill they learn in Recovering Together. They can reference these videos to learn new skills and to review skills from previous sessions. They will also have access to audio recordings, which will help the dyad practice the skills they learn.

The web resource accompanying Session 3 is:
- Distress Spiral Explainer Video

In the workbook, the content is presented as:

- What It Is
- How It Helps?
- When to Use It
- How to Use It

These sections can be delivered in any order based on your clinical judgment. Although we present scripts below, these are provided as examples. We encourage you to adapt to fit your style and the dyad's needs.

Agenda

Orient the dyad to Session 3 in their Workbooks. Remind them that the pictures represent the skills and new ones are added each week. Encourage them to practice and identify the ones that are most helpful.

Open your Workbooks to Session 3 (page 27). As a reminder, the pictures represent the skills from the prior and current sessions. These skills build on each other, and I encourage you to continue to try them all and see which work best for you.

Review the agenda with the dyad before checking in on the last session, skills practice, and any significant emotional distress or medical complications.

If you turn to page 30, you will see the agenda for today. We will review the skills discussed in the program so far and then discuss new skills. Today, we will be learning the skills of identifying your distress spiral and challenging unhelpful thoughts.

Check In and Review Prior Session and Prescription for Recovery (Home Practice)

Check in with the dyad to see how they are doing with the transition to rehab or home. Dyads typically look forward to being discharged from the hospital because it means that the patient is making good recovery. However, for many dyads the transition home can be challenging. Patients discharged to home and their caregivers may worry about being without constant medical attention. Patients and caregivers often notice that the old dynamics of relating to each other are no longer fitting because the patient continues to recover while the caregiver provides care on top of their regular responsibilities. There may be other family members and friends involved. Issues of challenges with communication may come up, and if they do, refer dyads to Session 4 for discussion the following week and continue to focus on the content of Session 3.

For dyads discharged to rehab, there might be disappointment about not going home and concerns about the recovery trajectory. Session 3 is a great opportunity to learn about these challenges and use them as you teach the skills of the distress spiral and challenging unhelpful thoughts.

Allowing space for dyads to catch you up to speed is helpful and will continue to enhance their engagement.

Thank you for being here today. How are you each doing today? How has the adjustment to home/rehab gone for each of you?

Briefly review the skills introduced in Sessions 1 and 2. Continue to explain and reinforce the value of home practice. Make a note from the last week about what they practiced, how they practiced, and what worked and what did not work, and use that information to individualize this skill review.

In our first two sessions, we discussed the skills of Deep Breathing, Mindful Stoplight, Staying in the 24-Hour Block, Mindfulness Meditation, Dialectics, and Hands as Worries. Practicing the skills regularly (not only when you are stressed) helps them become second nature. The more we practice, the easier the skills will be to access when you are feeling stressed. Last week you shared that [add specifics about what they practiced, if they practiced, which skills they liked].

Ask the dyad if they were able to practice skills. Discuss ways that they practiced.

What skills did you practice this week? How did that go?

If the dyad practiced any skills, validate their practice. Explore how they practiced and which skills they used. Compare and contrast with how they did the previous week. Ask whether they noticed any changes after using the skills.

That's amazing! Which skills did you practice? When did you use them? Did you practice individually or together? Did you notice any change after?

If the dyad did not practice, validate the challenges of practicing. Reiterate the value of practice.

It is sometimes hard to practice when you move from the hospital to rehab or home. Your schedules are different now. Let's problem-solve together how to make skill practice part of your routine.

Help them problem-solve their reported barriers. If they did not understand a skill, explain it again. Use the "Be Strategic" section (Workbook page 30) to create a plan to practice. Reinforce the plan at the end of the session. Review the tips for and value of practicing together. Often dyads feel that they "don't have time." Problem-solve how to incorporate skill practice within their routines.

How can we help you practice? When can you practice? Where can you do it? How can you incorporate practice into your daily routine?

Practicing the skills together is a valuable way to hold each other accountable. You can remind each other and integrate the skills into a routine (such as listening to a meditation at night). What are some ways that you can practice together or help remind each other?

Skills (Teach and Practice)

Identifying the Distress Spiral

Introduce the ANI as a stressor that can trigger negative thoughts, unhelpful behaviors, and unpleasant emotions. It is important to discuss how these are automatic (we don't choose them), and sometimes we are not even aware of what we are thinking or feeling, or why we are doing or not doing certain behaviors. Ask each partner to give examples of negative thoughts, behaviors, and emotions.

In the first skill for today you will learn to understand your and your partner's stressors. The acute neurological event is a tremendous stressor that automatically triggers negative thoughts, unhelpful behaviors, and unpleasant emotions. Many times the negative thoughts are about the past, the future, yourself, your partner, or extended family or friends. What kinds of negative thoughts have you noticed?

Unhelpful behaviors can be not following recommendations from the medical team, not eating, not sleeping, avoiding friends, and lashing out. What kinds of unhelpful behaviors have you noticed?

Unpleasant emotions can be sadness, panic, feeling frightened, or feeling depressed. What unpleasant emotions have you noticed?

If they have trouble responding, ask them to help each other based on what they have noticed. You can also use their responses on the HADS and PCL. Validate their responses even when not accurate and reshape as needed.

> *Sometimes it is hard to think of specific thoughts, behaviors, or emotions. Would it be OK if your partner helps us out with an example based on what they observed? Let's take a look at your answers to the assessments to see if we can find some clues.*

Once the patient and caregiver are able to identify thoughts, behaviors, and emotions, introduce the Distress Spiral (page 31 in the Workbook). Explain how the ANI is an incredibly challenging experience that can place the dyad on the Distress Spiral. Check in with the dyad to ensure that they understand the concept.

> *Negative thoughts, unpleasant emotions, and unhelpful behaviors are interrelated. This means that they feed off each other and make each other worse over time. You can think of this as a snowball of negativity that gets bigger and bigger over time. We call this the Distress Spiral. The Distress Spiral is triggered by stressful events. The ANI experience is particularly stressful and challenging and can place you and your loved one on the Distress Spiral. What do you think about the Distress Spiral?*

If the exercise does not resonate with them, reassure them that you will discuss examples later in the session and things will become more clear.

> *Being aware and curious about your negative thoughts, unpleasant emotions, and unhelpful behaviors is really important. Once you identify these, you have the opportunity to move toward the Emotional Recovery Path. Because the thoughts, emotions, and behaviors are automatic, sometimes it is easier to recognize them in your partner than in yourself. You can help each other by sharing what you notice about your own thoughts, behaviors, and emotions, and what you notice about your partner. The Observe and Describe components of the Mindful Stoplight can help you become aware of your thoughts, emotions, and behaviors.*

Discuss strategies to move toward the Emotional Recovery Path by using the program skills. Next orient the dyad to the diagram on page 32 of the Workbook, and review the example.

You can move from the Distress Spiral to the Emotional Recovery Path by using the skills in the Recovering Together toolkit. Let's turn to page 32 in your Workbook, which shows an example of the Distress Spiral on the left and the Emotional Recovery Path on the right. What thoughts, emotions, or behaviors from the left side resonate with you? How about from the right side?

Guide the dyads to complete their own Distress Spiral and Emotional Recovery Path. Help them as needed by using what you've learned about them thus far. Validate and encourage them.

Now let's turn to page 33 in your Workbook. We will create your own Distress Spiral and Emotional Recovery Path. Let's start with the Distress Spiral on the left. Write down negative thoughts, unpleasant emotions, and unhelpful behaviors.

Now let's work on the right side, the Emotional Recovery Path. What behaviors do you think would help you? What thoughts? Many times changing the behaviors and thoughts will lead to more pleasant emotions.

Once they each create their personal Distress Spiral and Emotional Recovery Path, help the dyads understand that the Distress Spiral negatively impacts their physical health and their recovery. Help them understand that their spirals are interrelated as dyads, and that one person's thoughts, behaviors, and emotions impact the other's. This is why it is important for them to work together and help each other. Ensure that the caregiver is being open about their own challenges and not overfocusing on the patient. If this occurs, gently point it out and discuss that their Emotional Recovery Path impacts that of their loved one.

How do you think the Distress Spiral impacts physical recovery and overall health?

How can you use the Recovering Together toolkit to move toward the Emotional Recovery Path?

How can you be open to your experiences and communicate them to your partner?

Validate their experiences. Share how the communication module may be helpful and offer to conduct it during next session.

Challenging Unhelpful Thoughts After ANI

Describe how they identify thoughts using with Mindful Stoplight skills (Observe and Describe), they have the opportunity to engage with the last step of mindfulness (Act with Awareness) and investigate whether the thoughts are based on facts or not. Help the dyad understand that most often our brains interpret negative thoughts as facts when in fact they are not. Ask the patient and caregiver for examples or share one yourself.

Earlier today we used the Mindful Stoplight skills of Observe and Describe to identify negative or unhelpful thoughts. Now that we have identified them, we can move to the last step of mindfulness, which is to Act with Awareness. This means that we can take an objective look at our thoughts and see if they are facts or perceptions. Most of the time our negative thoughts are not facts, but our brains perceive them as such. What do you think about this? Can you think of any negative thoughts that you might have thought were facts but later realized they were not?

If they don't agree or understand, validate and share how this is hard, and give examples. Next, explain why this skill is important. Help the dyad understand that reminding themselves that "thoughts are not facts" provides a reality check to the mind and helps the negative thoughts fade away, allowing us to move toward the Emotional Recovery Path. Here you can also remind them that Hands as Worries is another way to get distance from negative thoughts.

The simple act of reminding yourself that "Thoughts are not facts" makes the thoughts fade into the background. You may immediately feel better and more motivated to do things you enjoy or need to do for your recovery. It is truly a powerful process to watch the thoughts fade as you make the choice that they are not true or important. In this way you can move toward the Emotional Recovery Path.

Also, remember the Hands as Worries skill we learned last week. You can use that skill to help you get distance from negative thoughts. Regardless of which skill you use or which works best for you, the most important thing is to get distance from unhelpful thoughts so that they don't negatively affect your emotional recovery.

Ask the dyad for their impressions.

What do each of you think about this? When might this skill of Challenging Unhelpful Thoughts be useful?

Discuss when to use this skill.

You can use this skill when you notice unhelpful thoughts. You can also help each other when you hear one another speak and notice unhelpful thoughts. You can remind each other that "Thoughts are not facts."

Discuss how the patient and caregiver can help each other move toward the Emotional Recovery Path. Encourage them to review the Distress Spiral Explainer Video on the website, which can be accessed by searching for this book's title on the Oxford Academic platform at academic.oup.com.

Working together and supporting each other in the recovery process is so important. There are many ways you can do this. You can be honest with your partner and share how you are feeling. You can express that you are on their side. You can help give them perspective when they are caught on the Distress Spiral. Listen to each other and give one another the opportunity to communicate about what really bothers you. Plan together for which skills would be most helpful. When you receive support, let your partner know that you appreciate their response and help.

Session 3 Summary

Orient the patient and caregiver to the summary and table of skills at the end of Session 3 in the Workbook. Briefly review the session content and skills.

On pages 34–35 in your Workbooks, there is a summary of our session. This table is a great way to quickly reference skills. Today, we learned about the benefits of identifying the Distress Spiral and how to move toward the Emotional Recovery Path. We discussed how to identify that thoughts are not facts how to challenge unhelpful or negative thoughts after ANI. Throughout the session we also discussed how to support each other.

Ask the dyad which skill(s) they want to practice over the next week. Explore how they might build on the skills they learned in prior sessions.

So far, which skills do you like the best? Which ones will be most useful over the next week?

Prescription for Recovery (Home Practice)

Remind the dyad about the weekly Prescription for Recovery section. Ask for specific times that they will plan to use the skills.

As we go along, the Prescription for Recovery is a helpful reminder to practice the skills, including those from prior sessions (Deep Breathing, Mindful Stoplight, Staying in the 24-Hour Block, Mindfulness Meditation, Dialectics, and Hands as Worries) and the new ones from today (Identifying the Distress Spiral and Challenging Unhelpful Thoughts). You can take notes about skills to practice, goals for your practice for skills, and any questions that come up between sessions. Do you have ideas of how you can apply the skills over the next week?

When appropriate, encourage the patient and caregiver to keep each other accountable with practice. Remind them that practice is flexible, and they can do it anywhere and anytime.

It can be helpful to plan times to practice together (or individually). That way, you can help hold each other accountable. Remember, you can practice the skills anytime and anywhere—the goal is to make them a part of everyday life.

Remind the dyad to practice skills using materials they can access by searching for this book's title on the Oxford Academic platform at academic.oup.com.

Remember that the website can facilitate practice. We created recordings that can be accessed by searching for this book's title on the Oxford Academic platform at academic.oup.com.

Schedule Next Session

Schedule the session for next week.

When works for you both next week?

End the session by thanking the dyad for their participation. Answer their questions and remind them that they will receive an email to complete the measures prior to the next session.

Thank you for your participation today! Do you have any final questions? Feel free to email or call me if anything changes or you need anything. Also, before the next session, you will receive an email from me to complete the same measures prior to the next session. This helps me understand how you are each doing and tailor the program accordingly. I'll see you on [DATE] and [TIME], and please reach out at any point.

CHAPTER 4

Session 4: Navigating Relationships

(Corresponds to Session 4 of the Workbook)

Materials

- Clinician Guide and Workbooks
- Pens

Outline of Session 4

Session 4 Goals

Preparing for Session 4

- Recommendations for Clinicians
- Logistics for Delivery
- Assessment (administer and/or review measures of depression, anxiety, and posttraumatic stress for each dyad member)

Session 4

Agenda

Check In and Review Prior Session and Prescription for Recovery (Home Practice)

Skills (Teach and Practice)

- Education
- Effective Communication

Session 4 Summary

Prescription for Recovery (Home Practice)

Schedule Next Session

1. Continue to build rapport with the dyad and validate their experiences. If home practice is not a habit yet, encourage them to integrate into daily life.
2. Continue allowing flexibility with scheduling.
3. Teach skills by applying them to the individual challenges of the dyad. Focus on experiential learning and encourage the patient and caregiver to come up with their own examples. This session is focused on communication, and it is important to take a strengths-based dyadic approach, which is different from couples or family therapy. Enhancing communication and priotizing the relationship are key goals of this session.

Preparing for Session 4

Recommendations for Clinicians

In this session it is important to continue to build and maintain rapport with each member of the dyad by using a strengths-based dyadic approach. The goal of this session is to focus on how the two partners communicate and how they can use the skills to improve their communication. Do your best to highlight the positive aspects of the dyadic interpersonal style (e.g., cooperation, dedication) and deliver practical skills for handling the emotional distress/stress of managing the ANI aftermath together. As the clinician, ask yourself, "Am I focusing on the relationship or the dyad's response to the stressor/ANI?" This is a subtle consideration for this session. We will want to preserve the relationship or even enhance it, but the focus should be on their reaction to and coping with ANI, rather than other life events or situations that they might bring to the session.

Dyads will enter this session with various agendas and ways of communicating. By now, you will likely be aware of their patterns of communication and things you have learned or observed in prior sessions together. If the dyad did not have a close or healthy relationship before the ANI, things will likely come up in this session. It is important to redirect the dyad to the goal of this session, which is communication in the context of the ANI. Communication about the overall quality of the relationship or things from the past is not helpful in the context of a brief intervention, can deter from recovery after the ANI, and can cause further deterioration in the relationship. Couples can be referred to couples therapy, and other types of dyads can be referred to family or other forms of therapy to specifically target the relationship quality. By validating and focusing on each individual's strength you can gently move the dyad toward learning how to communicate about their needs in the context of recovery after the ANI. At the same time, if the dyad comes in with a good relationship, it is important to preserve the quality of the relationship while helping them manage the ANI together.

As mentioned in prior sessions, adapt the material however you see fit. Although we provide scripts throughout the session, they are only examples. It is most important to be authentic to your clinical style. This session is meant to be flexible, as long as you deliver the program skills.

Logistics for Delivery

The patient and caregiver may or may not be together, so they might access the session from the same device or different devices. Location should not impact treatment as long as both patient and caregiver are engaged.

Assessment

Prior to the session, review each dyad member's responses to the validated measures of depression and anxiety (Hospital Anxiety and Depression Scale [HADS]) and posttraumatic stress (Posttraumatic Stress Disorder Checklist for DSM-5 [PCL-5]) (see Introduction for details on assessments). You can send the measures over email prior to each session or have the dyad complete them at the beginning of each session. Regular assessment of symptoms allows you to track progress and tailor the skills to help address specific symptoms.

The measures are also included on pages 38–39 of the Workbook. The items of these measures correspond to symptoms. Reviewing them informs how to tailor the content to address the dyad's needs. For example, on the HADS, if they endorse more anxiety symptoms such as feeling "tense or wound up," then explain how Deep Breathing can help reduce physiological arousal. You can also spend more time on skills that are most relevant to their current distress because this will facilitate home practice. You can also use the symptoms they endorse on the measures as examples when explaining skills.

Session 4

The rest of this chapter aligns with Session 4 in the workbook. Refer the dyad to page 37 in their Workbook. By searching for this book's title on the Oxford Academic platform at academic.oup.com, the dyad will have access to explainer videos pertaining to each skill they will learn in Recovering Together. They can reference these videos to learn new skills and to review skills learned in previous sessions. They will also have access to audio recordings, which will help them practice the skills they learn.

The web resource accompanying Session 4 is:

■ Effective Communication Explainer Video

In the workbook, the content is presented as:

■ What It Is
■ How It Helps
■ When to Use It
■ How to Use It

These sections can be delivered in any order based on your clinical judgment. Although we present scripts below, these are provided as examples. We encourage you to adapt them to fit your style and the dyad's needs.

Agenda

Orient the dyad to Session 4 in their Workbooks. Remind them that the pictures represent the skills and new ones are added each week. Encourage them to practice and identify the ones that are most helpful.

Open your Workbooks to Session 4 (page 37). As a reminder, the pictures represent the skills from the prior and current sessions. These skills build on each other, and I encourage you to continue to try them all and see which work best for you.

Review the agenda with the dyad before checking in on the last session, skills practice, and any significant emotional distress or medical complications.

If you turn to page 40, you will see the agenda for today. We will review the materials discussed over the course of the program so far and then discuss new skills. Today, we will be learning the skills of Effective Communication.

Check In and Review Prior Session and Prescription for Recovery (Home Practice)

Check in with the dyad to see how they are doing. By now the dyad should be adjusted to home or rehab and the patient should be even more engaged and active.

Thank you for being here today. How are you each doing today? How has the past week gone for each of you?

Briefly review the skills introduced in the previous session and prior sessions. Continue to explain and reinforce the value of home practice. Reinforce every practice they did. Reiterate that the goal is to incorporate home practice in their daily lives. Make a note from the last week about what they practiced, how they practiced, and what worked and did not work, and use that information to individualize this skill review. (Base what you say next on the actual skills covered. Since this is a modular treatment, following Sessions 1 and 2 the dyad and you will have selected specific sessions to focus on, and therefore not all the listed skills will have been learned).

In our prior sessions, we discussed the skills of [Deep Breathing, Mindful Stoplight, Staying in the 24-Hour Block, Mindfulness Meditation, Dialectics, Hands as Worries, Identifying the Distress Spiral, and Challenging Unhelpful Thoughts]. Practicing the skills regularly (not only when you are stressed) helps them become second nature. Incorporating the skills into your daily routine and reminding each other to practice will help practicing become habit. Last week you shared that [add specifics about what they practiced, if they practiced, and which skills they liked].

Ask the dyad if they were able to practice skills. Discuss ways that they practiced.

What skills did you practice this week? How did that go?

If the dyad practiced any skills, validate their practice. Explore how they practiced and which skills they used. Compare and contrast with how they did the previous week. Ask whether they noticed any changes after using the skills.

That's amazing! Which skills did you practice? When did you use them? Did you practice individually or together? Did you notice any change after?

If the dyad did not practice, validate the challenges of practicing. Reiterate the value of practice.

It is sometimes hard to practice when you move from the hospital to rehab or home. Your schedules are different now. Let's problem-solve together how to make skill practice part of your routine.

Help them problem-solve their reported barriers. If they did not understand a skill, explain it again. Use the "Be Strategic" section (Workbook page 40) to create a plan to practice. Reinforce the plan at the end of the session. Review the tips for and value of practicing together. Often dyads feel that they "don't have time." Problem-solve how to incorporate skill practice within their routines. Make sure they know that any practice is better than no practice.

How can we help you practice? When can you practice? Where can you do it? How can you incorporate practice into your daily routine?

Practicing the skills together is a valuable way to hold each other accountable. You can remind each other and integrate the skills into a routine (such as listening to a meditation at night). What are some ways that you can practice together or help remind each other?

Life can get in the way and sometimes we can't practice as much as we'd like to. Any home practice is better than no practice. What are easy ways to practice regardless of how busy you are? How can you incorporate practice into your daily routine?

Skills (Teach and Practice)

Education

Provide education on the importance of communication. Emphasize that communication challenges are normal during times of stress and transition. Validate the dyad's effort in participating in the program together. Share that communication is all about listening to each other and sharing. You can describe this session as "passing the ball back and forth."

Today we will learn about Effective Communication. Communication is essential to relationships. Communicating about thoughts, feelings, and experiences—especially during times of stress—is not easy. Sometimes we have the tendency to stray away from communicating in times of stress because we: (1) don't know how to, (2) worry about our partner's response, and (3) have perceptions about how the other person will respond that sometimes are not true. Good communication brings people closer together. Because stress can make communication more challenging, and the ANI stress can bring up new emotions and change existing roles, learning Effective Communication skills is vital. Expressing your needs and actively listening to your loved one can help you preserve roles and work together as a team. Sharing needs will bring back a sense of normalcy. Communication is key to understanding and sharing your individual experiences with ANI (your thoughts, emotions, experiences, and roles).

Dialectics and mindfulness are very helpful in communicating with each other. Can you use the Mindful Stoplight (see Session 1) and, with curiosity, Observe and Describe what your life with your partner was like before the ANI? What about what it is like now, in this moment? What has changed? What has stayed the same?

If the dyad has trouble, ask them to help each other based on what they noticed. Elicit previous roles the dyad served for each other and in their social sphere and attempt to juxtapose these on current circumstances. The illustration on Workbook page 42 can be helpful as an example.

Sometimes it is hard to think of specific situations. Would it be OK if your partner helps us out with an example based on what they have observed?

So it sounds like you were the _____ for the two of you and now you are _____. How does that feel?

Effective Communication

In this section it is important to stress the shift to a "We-focus" versus an "I-focus" or a "You-focus." Problems are "We-problems" that are navigated best together, and solutions are "We-solutions." Emphasize that the patient and caregiver can remind each other by asking, "How can we navigate this together?"

Effective Communication involves expressing your thoughts, feelings, needs, and preferences and being receptive to your loved one's. In relationships, both individual and shared experiences have value. The tendency to avoid sharing difficult thoughts and emotions is normal, but it can increase stress. This stress can spill over into interactions and lead to hurt feelings, guilt, and conflict. Expressing thoughts, feelings, and needs in specific, clear ways and listening without judgment to your loved one's can help you understand each other. It can help you focus on individual and shared challenges as "We-problems." This will help restore balance in your relationship and maintain closeness. Together you can plan and solve problems, and understand one another as a team.

Help dyads understand when to use Effective Communication, including sharing how they feel and what they need. Teach dyads the importance of using the skills in their Recovering Together skills to regulate their emotions before, during, and after conversations. Help them understand that heightened emotions can get in the way of being able to fully listen and effectively communicate.

In order to communicate effectively with each other it is important to keep your emotions in check and regulate them before, during, and after the conversation. Doing so will allow you to be able to fully listen, be present, and respond in a helpful way to your partner. What skills in your Recovering Together toolkit can you use to regulate your emotions?

If dyads have trouble, point them to Deep Breathing, Dialectics, and the Mindful Stoplight. Validate and encourage them. Next, you can share the steps for Effective Communication. Also, remind them that they can review the Effective Communication Explainer Video by searching for this book's title on the Oxford Academic platform at academic.oup.com.

We created a roadmap that breaks down communication into several steps that we will practice today. The steps are (1) clarify your goals, (2) practice Mindful Stoplight skills, (3) Challenge Unhelpful Thoughts, (4) use Dialectics, and (5) Act with Awareness.

Before Conversations

Turn to page 43 in the Workbook, and go through the exercise together. Be intentional about which topics to discuss. Make sure that the topics align with the recovery after ANI. The dyad can pick topics that are important for both to discuss and those that they have been avoiding. If they have trouble generating topics, you can also ask them to think of any topics that are easy to talk about and others that are harder.

Let's brainstorm about what topics you would like to discuss with each other. What do you think it would be important for you both to talk about?

If they have trouble, you can make suggestions based on what you have observed over the past few sessions. It is important for both of them to want to discuss the topic.

Now that we have a topic, let's clarify the goals of the conversation. Goals will help us stay focused and avoid misunderstandings or conflict. Conversations can have more than one goal. If there are multiple goals, it is important to balance them. Ask yourself three questions:

1. *What do I want to achieve with this conversation?*
2. *What do I want my relationship with this person to look like after this conversation?*
3. *How do I want to feel about myself when I am done with this conversation?*

Once you answer these questions, you can think through what is more important: getting what you want, preserving the relationship, or feeling good about how you handled the situation.

Help the patient and caregiver understand (with examples) how—depending on the situation—one, two, or all goals are important.

As you can imagine, it may not always be necessary to satisfy all three goals. If I am at the grocery store and the cashier is being rude, it may only be important that I complete my first goal—getting the groceries. At the doctor's office, it may be important to maintain a good working relationship versus getting what you want. In your relationship to one another, it may be most important to preserve self-respect and integrity along with your relationship.

Sometimes you satisfy one or more goals, and sometimes you don't, so stay flexible. Does this make sense to you two?

Ask the dyad for examples of conversations where they might think about their goals. They should write these down at the end of Step 1 in their Workbooks on page 44. Next move to Step 2: Practice Mindful Stoplight Skills. Make sure the dyad has a good grasp of these skills, and ask them if they use them and how. Ask the dyad for examples or use examples that they have shared in the past. Remind the dyad that "thoughts are not facts" and to notice anything that comes up that is unhelpful or puts them on the Distress Spiral. If you did not cover Session 3, then briefly explain the concept of "thoughts and feelings are not facts" as it is important for this session. Note that they can read more about it in Session 3.

Great! Now that we have a topic and goals, let's move to Step 2. Here we practice the Mindful Stoplight to understand what we are feeling and regulate emotions. Here we are using Mindful Stoplight skills. Have you used these before? Let's Observe and Describe thoughts and feelings related to this particular topic of conversation. Remember that thoughts are not facts, and that it is important to be curious about your experiences and nonjudgmental.

If the dyad has trouble, help them using what you have learned from them in prior sessions. Make sure you validate and there is agreement.

Next, move to Step 3: Challenge Unhelpful Thoughts. Help them catch any judgments or assumptions, and whether these are related to their own or their partner's experiences. Help the patient and caregiver remember that thoughts are not facts, and that no thought is inherently good or bad.

> *Great! Now let's think about any judgments or assumptions you might both have about yourself or your partner's experiences. Remember that "thoughts are not facts," and it is important to challenge assumptions or judgments as a team to promote emotional recovery. Can you identify any judgments or assumptions? How might you change those?*

Often dyads are less able to see their own assumptions or judgments and are better able to identify those of their partner. Validate this experience. Help them ask questions to get to more accurate thoughts. The next step is to help them use Dialectics to see that they can have more than one thought, more than one feeling about the experience. Remind them what Dialectics are. Use as many examples as you need.

> *The next step is to use Dialectics. Do you remember Dialectics? What are they? Yes, Dialectics means that more than one thought or emotion can be true at the same time, so you do not need to choose one of them. In other words, you can have multiple perspectives, sometimes different, about your relationship or situation, and they all can be true. Read the examples on page 44 of your Workbook. Can you identify the Dialectics related to your relationship?*

Then the next step is Acting with Awareness. Emphasize using skills learned so far in the program: Mindful Stoplight, Deep Breathing, Dialectics, acceptance, noticing the partner's stressors, identifying goals of conversation, and using skills in times of stress.

> *Finally, Act with Awareness. Deep Breathing and mindfulness skills can help you regulate your emotions so you can Act with Awareness. Think about what other skills you might be able to use to help you feel relaxed before conversations. What might be the best times and places to have challenging conversations? For some people, that is at the end of the day, or Sunday afternoon, or while taking a walk. What works for you?*

Make sure dyads understand the importance of using skills to set the stage for Effective Communication. Use Mindful Stoplight skills to think about ways to Act with Awareness, mindfulness/relaxation to regulate emotions, and Act with Awareness to be intentional about conversations.

During Conversations

Discuss how the skills in the Recovering Together toolkit also help us stay open, present, and engaged during conversations. Next, review the tips for expressing needs, listening to loved ones, and tips for both patient and caregiver, and ask them to circle any examples what worked for them or to add new suggestions. Discuss the role of tone of voice and body language in maintaining calm, and how the dyad can support each other if they notice that one of them might be on a Distress Spiral. Discuss the concepts of "mini-breaks" and how these can be used by one or both partners to get some space and regulate emotions before returning to the conversation.

On page 45 of your Workbook, there are tips for expressing needs. How might you use mindfulness, Dialectics, and "thoughts are not facts" to support you with expressing your needs? Can you give an example?

On page 45 of your Workbook, there are tips for listening to your loved one's needs. What resonates for you on the page?

On page 46 of your Workbook, there are tips for both of you, including the use of "mini-breaks." Mini breaks are helpful when you notice increased emotions in you or your partner that interfere with a productive conversation. You and your partner can decide to stop the conversation, use skills from your Recovering Together toolkit, and then return to finish the conversation at a different time. What do you think about using mini-breaks?

After Conversations

Discuss how the Recovering Together skills also help us regulate emotions. Help the dyad see that the same skills apply to both situations.

Help them understand that this is important because often emotions increase at the end of the conversation, and relaxing after conversations will help keep "fuel in the tank" for future discussions and help them continue to work as a team.

Often emotions get stronger after the conversation. You can use the same skills to Observe and Describe emotions, check judgments or misconceptions, and help each other stay relaxed. Evaluate how the conversation went, what you said, how you said it, and the solutions you identified. Remind yourself that Effective Communication is a skill that gets better with practice. Express appreciation to your partner and congratulate yourself, too. Find ways to help each other relax together or alone. Do something rewarding. What can you do to reward yourselves for communicating effectively? What can help regulate your emotions and ease your mind?

Help dyads come up with a plan. Deciding what to do can be a good opportunity to use skills.

Session 4 Summary

Orient the patient and caregiver to the summary and table of skills at the end of Session 4 in the workbook. Briefly review the session content and skills.

On page 47 in your Workbooks, there is a summary of our session. This table is a great way to quickly reference skills. Today, we learned that Effective Communication is important in relationships, especially during times of stress. We also discussed how mindfulness helps us notice and create space from emotions and thought to help regulate emotions. We discussed how Dialectics and "thoughts are not facts" can help, and how it is important to Act with Awareness.

Ask the dyad which skill(s) they want to practice over the next week. Explore how they might build on the skills they learned in prior sessions. Encourage them to use Effective Communication strategies in their day-to-day communication or to discuss additional topics that they have been avoiding.

So far, which skills do you like the best? Which ones will be most useful over the next week? Can you try incorporating Effective Communication skills in ways you talk with each other?

Prescription for Recovery (Home Practice)

Remind the dyad about the weekly Prescription for Recovery section. Ask for specific times that they will plan to use the skills. (Base what you say next on the actual skills covered. Since this is a modular treatment, following Sessions 1 and 2 the dyad and you will have selected specific sessions to focus on and therefore not all the listed skills will have been learned).

As we go along, the Prescription for Recovery continues to be a helpful reminder to practice the skills, including those from prior sessions [Deep Breathing, Mindful Stoplight, Staying in the 24-Hour block, Dialectics, Hands as Worries, Identifying the Distress Spiral, Challenging Unhelpful Thoughts] and the new one from today, Effective Communication. You can take notes about skills to practice, goals for your practice for skills, and any questions that come up between sessions. Do you have ideas of how you can apply the skills over the next week?

When appropriate, encourage the patient and caregiver to keep each other accountable with practice. Remind them that practice is flexible, and they can do it anywhere and anytime.

It can be helpful to plan times to practice together (or individually). That way, you can help hold each other accountable. Remember, you can practice the skills anytime and anywhere—the goal is to make them a part of everyday life.

Remind the dyad to practice skills using materials they can access by searching for this book's title on the Oxford Academic platform at academic.oup.com.

Remember that the website can help facilitate practice. We created recordings that can be accessed by searching for this book's title on the Oxford Academic platform at academic.oup.com.

Schedule the session for next week.

When works for you both next week?

End the session by thanking the dyad for their participation. Answer their questions and remind them that they will receive an email to complete the measures prior to the next session.

Thank you for your participation today! Do you have any final questions? Feel free to email or call me if anything changes or you need anything. Also, before the next session, you will receive an email from me to complete the same measures prior to the next session. This helps me understand how you are each doing and tailor the program accordingly. I'll see you on [DATE] and [TIME], and please reach out at any point.

CHAPTER 5

Session 5: Engaging with Positive Activities

(Corresponds to Session 5 of the Workbook)

Materials

- Clinician Guide and Workbooks
- Pens

Outline of Session 5

Session 5 Goals

Preparing for Session 5

    Recommendations for Clinicians

    Logistics for Delivery

    Assessment (administer and/or review measures of depression, anxiety, and posttraumatic stress for each dyad member)

Session 5

Agenda

Check In and Review Prior Session and Prescription for Recovery (Home Practice)

Skills (Teach and Practice)

- Behavioral Activation
- Social Support
- Daily Goals

Session 5 Summary

Prescription for Recovery (Home Practice)

Schedule Next Session

1. This session is geared toward patients and/or caregivers with elevated depression scores (on the Hospital Anxiety and Depression Scale [HADS]). These symptoms can be difficult to change quickly. Model flexibility, curiosity, and lack of judgment as you discuss challenges in practicing or engaging in activities.

2. Tailor the content to the dyad. Encourage the patient and caregiver to identify activities that have been helpful in the past or are important to them now. Use Socratic questioning to help them guide the conversation. Help them problem-solve barriers to engaging in activities and with social networks. The goal is to make the content applicable to their daily lives.

3. Use a strengths-based approach. The patient and/or caregiver will likely be experiencing mild to moderate depressive symptoms. Highlight the activities and social supports they are already using. Be encouraging and empower them to make small behavioral changes to move toward goals and values.

Preparing for Session 5

Recommendations for Clinicians

The therapeutic alliance continues to be important for program engagement and completion. Consistent with prior sessions, explain skills clearly and as simply as possible. (Remember that all dyads receive Sessions 1 and 2 and then pick four of the remaining five sessions with the clinician's guidance). This session is best for dyads with elevated depression scores (on the HADS assessment). If they endorse primarily anxiety symptoms (and minimal depressive symptoms), then you may recommend Session 6, Managing Fear and Worries, instead. If the dyad scores high on both, then they may opt to do Sessions 5 and 6 and skip a different one.

Adapt the material however you see fit. Although we provide scripts throughout the session, they are only examples. It is most important to be authentic to your clinical style. This session is meant to be flexible, as long as you deliver the program skills.

Logistics for Delivery

Session 5 is typically delivered over live video (e.g., Zoom). Dyads are usually home by now, although some patients may be in a rehabilitation center or even rehospitalized. Adapt the delivery format to best meet the dyad's needs (in person, phone, live video).

Assessment

Prior to the session, review each dyad member's responses to the validated measures of depression and anxiety (HADS) and posttraumatic stress (Posttraumatic Stress Disorder Checklist for DSM-5 [PCL-5]) (see Introduction for details on assessments). You can send the measures over email prior to each session or have the dyad complete them at the beginning of each session. Regular assessment of symptoms allows you to track progress and tailor the skills to help address specific symptoms.

The measures are also included on pages 50–51 of the Workbook. The items of these measures correspond to symptoms. For this session, it is important to review the dyad's scores on the depression subscale and tailor the content accordingly.

Session 5

The rest of this chapter aligns with Session 5 in the workbook. Refer the dyad to page 49 in their Workbook. By searching for this book's title on the Oxford Academic platform at academic.oup.com, the dyad will have access to explainer videos pertaining to each skill they will learn in Recovering Together. They can reference these videos to learn new skills and to review skills learned in previous sessions. They will also have access to audio recordings, which will help them practice the skills they learn.

The web resource accompanying Session 5 is:

- Behavioral Activation Explainer Video

In the workbook, the content is presented as:

- What It Is
- How It Helps
- When to Use It
- How to Use It

These sections can be delivered in any order based on your clinical judgment. Although we present scripts below, these are provided as examples. We encourage you to adapt to fit your style and the dyad's needs.

Agenda

Orient the dyad to Session 5 in their Workbooks. Remind them that the pictures represent the skills and new ones are added each week. Encourage them to identify ones that are most helpful.

Open your Workbooks to Session 5 (page 49). You'll see the pictures of the skills from prior sessions and this session. Experiment with them and see which work best for you. They also can be used together.

Review the agenda with the dyad before checking in on the last session, skills practice, and any significant emotional distress or medical complications.

On page 52, you will see the agenda for today. Today, we will be learning about Behavioral Activation, Social Support, and Daily Goals. All three skills are helpful for improving mood.

Check In and Review Prior Session and Prescription for Recovery (Home Practice)

Check in with the dyad to see how they are doing. Ask them about previously discussed skills and whether they have been practicing any of them.

How are you each doing since last week?

Have you been using any of the skills? How did that go? Which have you found to be helpful and when?

If the dyad did not practice, validate their experience and help them problem-solve barriers.

It is so hard to practice, especially with everything going on. The goal is to use skills in your daily lives so that they become "second nature." What do you think got in the way of practicing the skills? What would help you each practice?

Skills (Teach and Practice)

Behavioral Activation

Introduce Behavioral Activation.

Today we're going to use a skill that has been shown (with lots of evidence) to improve mood. This skill is called Behavioral Activation. Have you heard of this before? Basically, the goal is to engage with behaviors (activities or goals) that will help with your recovery.

Explain how behavioral changes can positively impact thoughts and emotions. Encourage use of prior skills such as Mindful Stoplight or Challenging Unhelpful Thoughts ("thoughts are not facts"). Explain that these strategies create distance from thoughts or emotions that may interfere with activities or goals. If you did not deliver Session 3, then briefly explain the concept of "thoughts and feelings are not facts" as it is important for this session. Note that they can read more about it in Session 3.

Often, we want to wait to feel better or motivated to do something. However, when we are sad or anxious or sick, we often don't feel like doing anything and therefore tend to avoid or withdraw. When we avoid or withdraw, this negatively impacts our mood.

So, the purpose of Behavioral Activation is to make a concrete plan to engage in both necessary and enjoyable activities. Of course, this can be hard when we feel sad or are stuck in negative spirals. In these cases, we can use our prior skills, such as Challenging Unhelpful Thoughts ("thoughts are not facts") from Session 3 or Mindful Stoplight from Session 1, to notice yet create distance from negative thoughts and feelings. It is important to remember that we do not need to do what thoughts and feelings tell us. We are bigger than them and can use skills to Observe and Describe them nonjudgmentally, since believing that they are the truth is not always helpful.

Behavioral Activation helps us to focus on tangible goals and meaningful activities, which then help improve our mood and thinking. In other words, what we do can change how we think and feel.

Explain that Behavioral Activation can be difficult, so encourage patient and caregiver to help each other practice it. Ask about activities that they each enjoy individually and together. Use the questions on page 54 of the Workbook to facilitate the discussion. Encourage the dyad to identify activities that help them improve their mood and relationship.

Have you ever noticed that some activities improve your mood? What are those activities for you? What are those activities for your loved one? What activities do you do together?

If the dyad has a good understanding of Dialectics, consider using it in session. Validate their engagement in activities, and gently challenge them to identify ways they can further engage or modify behaviors. As an example:

It is great that [patient] is moving more throughout the day, which is an important part of recovery. Is there anything about your current level of physical activity that you'd like to change or work toward in the future?

Orient the dyad to the table on page 54 in the Workbook. Explain that the table provides examples of activities that may be necessary and/or enjoyable. Encourage them to read through and identify any activities that may be helpful or relevant to them.

Now, turn to page 54 in your Workbooks. As you can see, there is a table of sample activities. These activities can be things that we have to do or things we like to do. Engaging in them can help us feel more productive, energized, and positive. Read through the list of activities. Do any stand out as being important or relevant to you? Which ones?

If any of the listed activities are of interest to the dyad, ask if any of these activities can be done together or separately. Encourage the patient and caregiver to come up with additional ideas.

You mentioned that [XXX] and [XXX] are things that you need to do or enjoy doing. Are these activities you do separately? Together?

What other activities do you need to do or enjoy doing—separately or together? When might you do them?

Encourage the dyad to review the Behavioral Activation Explainer Video by searching for this book's title on the Oxford Academic platform at academic.oup.com.

Social Support

Introduce Social Support as a skill. Explain how it can help us to engage in activities and enhance coping. Encourage patient and caregiver to think about people they can reach out to for support.

Although we have discussed activities that can be helpful for our lives and mood, it can still be hard to engage in them when we are tired or stressed. Using each other and our social networks can help hold ourselves accountable. Seeking support from our social networks can also help us cope and create a sense of normalcy. Knowing who to reach out to and how to reach out to them is important for our health and well-being.

Who are some people in your life that you can reach out to for support, or to engage in some of these activities we discussed?

Consider using the "magnifying glass" metaphor (described below in the script) to demonstrate how stressful events (such as an acute neurological illness [ANI]) can impact communication and relationships. Encourage patient and caregiver to use Effective Communication skills (if they covered it in Session 4).

Many times, people believe that after a devastating event like an ANI, everyone will band together. However, research suggests that an ANI can act as a magnifying glass for any existing strengths and vulnerabilities. Therefore, actively seeking out support and communicating effectively with others is key during this time.

If the dyad covered Session 4, then you can note:

In fact, the communication skills covered in Session 4 provide good insight into ways to engage with other. Do you remember those skills? I encourage you to review them again because they can be applied to all types of relationships.

Discuss the different types of Social Support. Assess how comfortable patient and caregiver feel seeking out different types of Social Support, and discuss strategies as needed.

Social Support can come in many different forms. We can ask our social networks for information, emotional support, validation, or belonging. [Expand on any or all of these depending on the dyad's reaction]. Reflect on who you can seek out for these various sources of support.

Do you feel comfortable seeking out support? How do you go about doing that?

Sometimes it means identifying the people who will be supportive and sharing your thoughts and feelings with them. To maintain that support system, it is important to express gratitude and appreciation to them.

Encourage patient and caregiver to think about how they can support one another. Share observations that you've noticed in session about how they have supported each other. It is important to validate their engagement in the program and practice of skills.

And what are some ways that you support each other during this time?

The fact that you've been participating in this program together demonstrates how you are gathering informational support and emotionally supporting each other. It has been very rewarding to watch you [give example of them supporting each other].

Daily Goals

Introduce the Daily Goals skill. Explain that this skill helps us engage in activities and with our social network.

The final skill for today is Daily Goals. As we've discussed, engaging in activities or with our social networks can be difficult when we feel sick or sad. Setting clear goals is a great strategy for accomplishing what we need. Goals can be set individually or together. They help us build sustainable habits that move us toward the life that we want to live.

Discuss how prior skills (Staying in the 24-Hour Block; Mindful Stoplight) can help set goals. Discuss strategies for setting goals. Emphasize the importance of making concrete goals and being kind (rather than critical) to ourselves and others, even if we do not meet the goal.

Some of our prior skills can help us set Daily Goals. Staying in the 24-Hour Block reminds us to focus on one goal for the day. The Mindful Stoplight (Observe and Describe) can also help us identify thoughts and feelings in the moment that may interfere with or promote goals. It is important to set manageable goals (one at a time) that are concrete and achievable. It is just as important to be nonjudgmental and kind to yourself and each other throughout the process.

Make sure to be conversational and gather the dyad's input and thoughts throughout. Identify a goal together in session (if you have time).

What are your reactions/thoughts? What might be difficult? What strategies might help you?

Can you each identify a Daily Goal for yourselves? What about a goal you can do together?

Session 5 Summary

Orient the patient and caregiver to the summary and table of skills at the end of Session 5 in the Workbook. Briefly review the session content and skills, and ask them which skill(s) may be helpful to use.

When you turn to page 57 in your Workbooks, just like at the end of other sessions, you'll see the summary of our session. Today, we discussed the importance of Behavioral Activation to enhance mood, activities that you can do together and individually, and how Social Support and Daily Goals can help with engagement. You can see the list of skills and when and how to use them. Do any of the skills stand out today as particularly helpful?

Prescription for Recovery (Home Practice)

Remind the dyad about the weekly Prescription for Recovery section. Ask for specific times that they will plan to use the skills.

For this next week, think about which skills you may use. Also remember that the website can facilitate practice. We created recordings that can be accessed by searching for this book's title on the Oxford Academic platform at academic.oup.com.

Schedule Next Session

Schedule the session for next week.

When works for you both next week?

End the session by thanking the dyad for their participation. Answer their questions and remind them that they will receive an email to complete the measures prior to the next session.

Thank you for your participation today! Do you have any final questions? Feel free to email or call me if anything changes or you need anything. Also, before the next session, you will receive an email from me to complete the same measures prior to the next session. This helps me understand how you are each doing and tailor the program accordingly. I'll see you on [DATE] and [TIME], and please reach out at any point.

CHAPTER 6

Session 6: Managing Fear and Worries

(Corresponds to Session 6 of the Workbook)

Materials

- Clinician Guide and Workbooks
- Pens

Outline of Session 6

Session 6 Goals

Preparing for Session 6

- Recommendations for Clinicians
- Logistics for Delivery
- Assessment (administer and/or review measures of depression, anxiety, and posttraumatic stress for each dyad member)

Session 6

Agenda

Check In and Review Prior Session and Prescription for Recovery (Home Practice)

Skills (Teach and Practice)

- Observing Fear and Worry
- Acceptance and Change (Dialectics)

Session 6 Summary

Prescription for Recovery (Home Practice)

Schedule Next Session

1. This session is geared toward patients and/or caregivers with elevated anxiety (on the Hospital Anxiety and Depression Scale [HADS]). Model flexibility, curiosity, and lack of judgment as you discuss anxiety, triggers, and challenges to home practice.
2. Tailor the content to the dyad. Use the HADS to guide which symptoms to target and encourage the dyad to identify their own examples throughout the session. Consider revisiting Mindful Stoplight and Dialectics skills or relevant thoughts/emotions discussed in prior sessions.
3. Normalize and validate the experience of fear and anxiety. Fear of recurrence is a common experience among patients with an acute neurological illness (ANI). Also, create a safe, calm therapeutic space. This session can be anxiety-provoking, so feel free to use prior skills as you see fit (e.g., Deep Breathing, mindfulness).

Preparing for Session 6

Recommendations for Clinicians

The therapeutic alliance continues to be important for engagement and completion. Explain skills clearly and as simply as possible. This session can resonate with dyads given that many fear an ANI will happen again. The fear and worry can be similar feelings to the uncertainty discussed in Session 2. Therefore, this session further extends Dialectics by focusing on the balance of acceptance and change.

This session is best for dyads with elevated anxiety scores (on the HADS). If the patient and/or caregiver become too emotionally activated during the session, practice mindfulness, Deep Breathing, and other skills in the Recovering Together toolkit to manage physical, cognitive, and emotional anxiety.

Adapt the material however you see fit. Although we provide scripts throughout the session, they are only examples. It is most important to be authentic to your clinical style. This session is meant to be flexible, as long as you deliver the program skills.

Logistics for Delivery

Session 6 is typically delivered over live video (e.g., Zoom). Dyads are usually home by now, although some patients may be in a rehabilitation center or even rehospitalized. Adapt the delivery format to best meet the dyad's needs (in-person, phone, live video).

Assessment

Prior to the session, review each dyad member's responses to the validated measures of depression and anxiety (HADS) and posttraumatic stress (Posttraumatic Stress Disorder Checklist for DSM-5 [PCL-5]) (see Introduction for details on assessments). You can send the measures over email prior to each session or have the dyad complete them at the beginning of each session. Regular assessment of symptoms allows you to track progress and tailor the skills to help address specific symptoms.

The measures are also included on pages 60–61 of the Workbook. The items of these measures correspond to symptoms. For this session, it is important to review the dyad's scores on the anxiety subscale and tailor the content accordingly.

Session 6

The rest of this chapter aligns with Session 6 in the Workbook. Refer the dyad to page 59 in their Workbook. By searching for this book's title on the Oxford Academic platform at academic.oup.com, the dyad will have access to explainer videos pertaining to each skill they will learn in Recovering Together. They can reference these videos to learn new skills and to review skills learned in previous sessions. They will also have access to audio recordings, which will help them practice the skills they learn.

The web resource accompanying Session 6 is:

- Acceptance and Change Explainer Video

In the Workbook, the content is presented as:

- What It Is
- How It Helps
- When to Use It
- How to Use It

These sections can be delivered in any order based on your clinical judgment. Although we present scripts below, these are provided as examples. We encourage you to adapt to fit your style and the dyad's needs.

Agenda

Orient the dyad to Session 6 in their Workbooks. Remind them that the pictures represent the skills and new ones are added each week. Encourage them to identify ones that are most helpful.

Open your Workbooks to session 6 (page 59). As you can see, pictures of the skills are displayed here. This is a visual reminder to try different skills in your toolkit.

Review the agenda with the dyad.

Today, we'll briefly review prior session skills. Then, we will discuss and practice mindfulness to observe fear and worry and learn the dialectic of acceptance and change. We will then review the weekly Prescription for Recovery.

Check In and Review Prior Session and Prescription for Recovery (Home Practice)

Check in with the dyad to see how they are doing. Ask them about previously discussed skills and whether they have been practicing any of them.

How have you each been doing since last week?

Have you been using any of the skills from your Recovering Together toolkit? How did that go? Which have you found to be helpful and when?

If the dyad did not practice, help them problem-solve barriers.

What do you think got in the way of practicing skills? What would help you each practice?

Skills (Teach and Practice)

Observing Fear and Worry

Provide psychoeducation about fear and worry. Inquire about the patient and caregiver's understanding and experience of them.

Fear and worries about the future are common after an acute neurological event. Today, we will talk about how they are different and ways to manage them. These strategies for identifying them and their triggers will help you become more aware of them. The goal is to be able to identify them, create distance from them, and live more in the present.

How do you each experience fear or worry? How are they different?

Explain the difference between fear and worry. Also, explain triggers and encourage dyads to share their individual and/or shared ones.

Fear is an emotion that helps protect us against a current or imagined threat. An imagined threat can happen during the day (memories) or at night (dreams). It is common among patients who experienced ANI and their loved ones. Things in our environment or our mind can trigger fear. These triggers are often benign (not harmful) on their own but can make us feel fearful—for example, anniversaries of the ANI, hearing about another ANI, or experiencing symptoms. For each of you, what do you think are your triggers?

On the other hand, worry is more related to our thinking. These thoughts try to protect us against future threat. Many people note that worrying makes them feel like they are "doing something." However, most of the time worrying is not helpful. It can increase avoidance, anxiety, and restlessness.

On pages 63–64 in your Workbook, you will see a chart that describes the difference between fear and worry. [Give them time to read through it]. Does the difference between them surprise you?

If the dyad has a hard time understanding the difference, that is fine. It is most important that they can identify triggers, fear, and worry. Encourage the dyad to use mindfulness to Observe and Describe fear and worry. Explain that noticing them requires being curious and avoiding judgment. If applicable, remind the dyad about the Hands as Worries skill (Session 2) and how we can let worries be there AND do not want them to interfere with our lives—which is when mindfulness can be helpful. Ask them to describe their experience in session.

Mindfulness helps us to Observe and Describe fear and worry with curiosity. Given that our anxious mind tend to be overly critical, using mindfulness can be helpful for creating distance from these thoughts and emotions. Also, remember the Hands as Worries skill? We can let our worries exist AND not want them to dictate how we behave. Mindfulness helps us label fear and worry without judgment, so we can choose how to move forward.

What do you usually do, feel, or think when you experience fear or worry?

Can you describe it to each other?

Normalize the patient's and caregiver's experience of fear and worries. Explain our "typical" approaches for controlling them and link to their description (if relevant). Encourage them to identify which of the myths are most relevant to them.

Yes, those are very common tendencies. Fear and worries are part of being human, yet we tend to either push worries away or ruminate on them (that is, think about them over and over). We also may criticize ourselves or even our loved ones for worrying. Review the myths on page 64 of the Workbook. These are some natural responses to fears and worries. Do any stand out as relevant to your experience?

Discuss the "How to Use It" section on page 65 in the Workbook. Read the bullet points if needed, but if this feels redundant, move through it more quickly. Explain that mindfulness allows us to acknowledge our experience and "buy time" before acting. Remind the dyad that "thoughts and emotions are not facts," and encourage them to help each other be curious in the moment. Orient them to the questions at the bottom of page 65 in the Workbook. Explain that these questions can facilitate practice.

Thank you both for sharing. Practicing mindfulness allows us to acknowledge thoughts and emotions without acting on them. And remember thoughts are not facts! Help each other be curious in the moment. Review the questions at the bottom of the page. These are things you can ask yourselves and each other to practice this skill of Observing Fear and Worry.

Acceptance and Change (Dialectics)

Introduce the skill of Acceptance and Change (Dialectics). Explain that they both can be helpful and how they are different. Explain that the patient and caregiver's use of acceptance and change may fluctuate over time (depending on where they are in their journey). Ask them to think of a dialectic (related to acceptance and change) that applies to them individually and together.

Now we are going to discuss the dialectic of acceptance and change. Using acceptance, change, or both can help you manage fear and worries. You will find that many things are in our control to change, while others are not. Therefore, these call for different actions—change, accept, or seek more information. It is important to stay mindful and flexibly consider new information when presented.

Acceptance helps us struggle less with what is already happening. It is useful when we don't have control over a situation. However, it does not mean liking it, giving up, or approving of it. Are there any examples you can think of that would be good to accept?

Change helps us move toward goals. It is useful when you can control things, even in an uncontrollable situation. You can help each other identify when there are things to change. Can you think of any examples?

Great, thanks for sharing. After an ANI, it can be hard to accept what happened AND make the changes required. This balance of acceptance and change also fluctuates throughout your journey. Early on, there may be more need for acceptance. Over time, there may be small changes you can each make to move toward recovery.

Where would you each say you are now? What have you learned to accept? What are you trying to change? See the table on page 67 in your Workbook for some examples.

Now, can you rephrase this as a dialectic? Are there any other examples? How does this dialectic apply to fear and worries?

Discuss how to practice acceptance. Explain it is helpful when coping with uncertainty. Demonstrate how mindfulness skills and Dialectics (from prior sessions) help promote acceptance. Ask the dyad to identify an example during the session.

Acceptance helps us tolerate things we cannot control. Because many things after an ANI are outside of your control, you've likely been using acceptance throughout the journey. We can practice acceptance through Mindful Stoplight and Dialectics skills. Let's practice right now.

First, we need to observe what we are thinking and feeling without judgment. See if you can identify that for yourselves.

If the thought or emotion is distressing, practice Deep Breathing or visualize an image that allows you to be present. For example, imagine you are in the water and pushing a beach ball under the water (those are your difficult thoughts and/or feelings). What do you think would happen? What if you let the beach ball float on the water while you swim toward what is important to you, such as each other? And if you have multiple thoughts or feelings, notice and label them. They can all be present.

Now, turn to page 68 in your Workbooks. Can you each share an example of a dialectic that you need to accept? You can write that down there.

Discuss how to practice change. Explain that there may be small things they can control, even in an uncertain time. Demonstrate how mindfulness and problem-solving can help them make changes. Ask them to identify an example. Try to have them outline the answers to the questions on page 68 in the Workbook. You can use the whiteboard function on Zoom or share your screen to write down responses. Give them time to practice acceptance and problem-solving in session. Guide them as needed and be clear about the steps. If you do not have time to practice in session, encourage the dyad to practice before the next session (fill out the Workbook together this week). Also, remind them that they can review the Acceptance and Change Explainer Video by searching for this book's title on the Oxford Academic platform at academic.oup.com.

Sometimes there are small things you can control after an ANI. In other words, there may be small changes you can make to move toward your goals and values. Mindfulness and problem-solving strategies help with that.

Now, can you each identify a thought or behavior that you can change—either together or separately? Can you each observe and describe it without judgment?

Great! Now, let's practice problem-solving. Turn to pages 68–69 in your Workbooks. Problem-solving involves breaking down your goal into smaller steps, identifying barriers, brainstorming solutions, and assessing outcomes.

What is your goal? Be as concrete and specific as possible.

What steps can you take to achieve that? Can you write one down for now?

What barriers may come up? Be as inclusive as possible. Barriers can be logistical, physical, or emotional. Write those down as well.

Can you each share your example?

Session 6 Summary

Orient the patient and caregiver to the summary and table of skills at the end of Session 6 in the Workbook. Briefly review the session content and skills and ask them when skill(s) may be helpful to use.

Turn to page 69 in your Workbooks to review a summary of our session. Today, we discussed Observing Fear and Worry and how Mindful Stoplight and Dialectics can help us manage them. We also discussed Acceptance and Change (Dialectics). We practiced both using prior skills. What do you each think of these skills? When might they be useful to use?

Prescription for Recovery (Home Practice)

Remind the dyad about the weekly Prescription for Recovery section. Ask for specific times that they will plan to use the skills.

I encourage you to practice these skills over the next week. Also remember that the website can facilitate practice. We created recordings that can be accessed by searching for this book's title on the Oxford Academic platform at academic.oup.com. Make note of when you use the skills and if/ how they are helpful.

Schedule Next Session

Schedule the session for next week (if this is not the final session).

When works for you both next week?

End the session by thanking the dyad for their participation. Answer their questions and remind them that they will receive an email to complete the measures prior to the next session.

Thank you for your participation today! Do you have any final questions? Feel free to email or call me if anything changes or you need anything. Also, before the next session, you will receive an email from me to complete the same measures prior to the next session. This helps me understand how you are each doing and tailor the program accordingly. I'll see you on [DATE] and [TIME], and please reach out at any point.

CHAPTER 7 — Session 7: Making Meaning

(Corresponds to Session 7 of the Workbook)

Materials

- Clinician Guide and Workbooks
- Pens

Outline of Session 7

Session 7 Goals

Preparing for Session 7
- Recommendations for Clinicians
- Logistics for Delivery
- Assessment (administer and/or review measures of depression, anxiety, and posttraumatic stress for each dyad member)

Session 7

Agenda

Check In and Review Prior Session and Prescription for Recovery (Home Practice)

Skills (Teach and Practice)

Making Meaning
- Using Reflection to Find Meaning
- Using Mindfulness to Find Meaning
- Dialectics
- Acceptance and Change

Summary of Session 7 and Entire Program

Prescription for Recovery (Home Practice)

End of Recovering Together Program

1. This is the last session of the program. It is important for the dyad members to celebrate their commitment to the program and investment in their shared recovery.
2. The content of this session relies heavily on prior skills. It is also an opportunity to weave in and review all program skills and how they might be used for Making Meaning.
3. Make sure the dyad members finish the session feeling good about their progress. If their symptoms have not improved, or if they determine that they have new goals (such as working more on their relationship), provide appropriate referrals. Similarly, if their scores on the Hospital Anxiety and Depression Scale (HADS] and the Posttraumatic Stress Disorder Checklist for DSM-5 (PCL-5) continue to be high, encourage additional treatment and offer referrals.

Preparing for Session 7

Recommendations for Clinicians

This is the last session of the program. The goal is for the dyad members to appreciate and reflect on their journey together and the skills they have learned. The session has only one skill, Making Meaning. Explain the skill clearly and as simply as possible.

This session can be cathartic. It is an opportunity to reorganize perceptions about the acute neurological illness (ANI) and, ideally, find something positive that came out of it. The positive aspects can be about oneself, one's partner, or the relationship. The ANI can also motivate further behavioral change. Make space for reflection when these issues come up.

The session brings back the skills of dialectics and mindfulness. However, feel free to stay open to other skills that the dyad might bring up, as well as suggest additional skills. Since this is the last session, it is also an opportunity to review all skills. Reinforce, as best you can, how the skills in the Recovering Together toolkit have a wide application, and encourage the dyad to be creative in using skills even after the program ends, and even outside the ANI experience.

Review the HADS and PCL scores and work on weaving responses into the session. Because this is the last session, if scores are elevated, it is important to discuss this issue with the dyad and make referrals.

It is possible that the patient's recovery has not gone as predicted and there are sequelae of the ANI. These concerns can come up in this session. Refer the dyad to medical care for any medical questions (as in all sessions). Use program skills to help the dyad members support each other and adjust.

Adapt the material however you see fit. Although we provide scripts throughout the session, they are only examples. It is most important to be authentic to your clinical style. This session is meant to be flexible, as long as you deliver the program skills.

Logistics for Delivery

Session 7 is typically delivered over live video (e.g., Zoom). Most dyads are home by now, although some patients may still be in a rehabilitation center or even rehospitalized. Adapt the delivery format to best meet the dyad's needs (in-person, phone, live video).

Assessment

Prior to the session, review each dyad member's responses to the validated measures of depression and anxiety (HADS) and posttraumatic stress (PCL-5) (see Introduction for details on assessments). You can send the measures over email prior to each session or have the dyad complete them at the beginning of each session. Regular assessment of symptoms allows you to track progress and tailor the skills to help address specific symptoms.

The measures are also included on pages 72–73 of the Workbook. The items of these measures correspond to symptoms. For this session, it is important to review all their scores and make recommendations for more care if necessary. It can also be helpful to compare scores of this session with their first scores and reflect on improvement/change.

The rest of this chapter aligns with Session 7 in the Workbook. Refer the dyad to page 71 in their Workbook. By searching for this book's title on the Oxford Academic platform at academic.oup.com, the dyad will have access to explainer videos pertaining to each skill they will learn in Recovering Together. They can reference these videos to learn new skills and to review skills learned in previous sessions. They will also have access to audio recordings, which will help them practice the skills.

The web resource accompanying Session 7 is:

- Making Meaning Explainer Video

In the workbook, the content is presented as:

- What Is It
- How It Helps
- When to Use It
- How to Use It

These sections can be delivered in any order based on your clinical judgment. Although we present scripts below, these are provided as examples. We encourage you to adapt to fit your style and the dyad's needs.

Agenda

Orient the dyad to Session 7 in their Workbooks. Remind them that the pictures represent the skills and new ones are added each week. Encourage them to identify ones that are most helpful.

Open your workbooks to Session 7 (page 71). As you can see, pictures of the skills are displayed here. This is a visual reminder to try different skills.

Review the agenda with the dyad.

Today, we will briefly review prior session skills. Then, we will discuss the value of Making Meaning for recovery. We will practice Making Meaning using reflections and Dialectics to find meaning. We will then review the weekly Prescription for Recovery. Since this is our last session together, we will also discuss how to continue practicing the program skills after the session ends.

Check In and Review Prior Session and Prescription for Recovery (Home Practice)

Check in with the dyad to see how they are doing. Ask them about previously discussed skills and whether they have been practicing any of them.

How have you each been doing since last week?

How are you feeling about this being the last session together?

Have you been using any of the skills from your Recovering Together toolkit? How did that go? Which have you found to be helpful and when?

If the dyad did not practice, help them problem-solve barriers.

What do you think got in the way of practicing skills? What would help you each practice?

Skills (Teach and Practice)

Making Meaning

Provide psychoeducation about Making Meaning. Assure the dyad that Making Meaning does not mean trying to find a reason for why the ANI happened (e.g., someone/something to blame). Rather, Making Meaning means forming an understanding of the trauma and the event that has taken place, and reflecting on the learning that has occurred as a result of it. Inquire about the patient and caregiver's understanding and experience of them.

Both of you have gone through a traumatic experience with the acute neurological illness, hospitalization, and rehabilitation. It is important to reflect on all aspects of this experience as a way to gain meaning. You may have similar or different experiences and reflections. We will make space for them all, because acknowledging and processing them can be powerful and healing. Processing these experiences can help us learn about ourselves and our loved ones.

What do you think about reflecting and Making Meaning?

Validate that Making Meaning means "leaning in" to experiences and thinking about the ANI and the challenges that the dyad has experienced and that there may be reluctance to engage in the process.

It can be challenging to reflect on the ANI because often thinking back on that experience brings fear and other negative emotions. It is in human nature to automatically avoid these experiences. Making Meaning skills help us face challenges by "leaning in" with the skills we already have, and processing experiences together. Processing allows us to reorganize difficult experiences so that they become less scary and overwhelming. However, Making Meaning requires time and intention. It may not happen overnight. We will start the conversation today, but you may need to continue having conversations together after the program ends. For each of you, what do you think about the importance of reflecting on and Making Meaning of your experience with the acute neurological illness?

Making Meaning boils down to reflection, mindfulness, and dialectics. Reflections can help us process and accept our experiences and our loved one's experiences. Reflection helps us think back on past experiences with new perspectives, as observers. Mindfulness can help us make room for reactions and emotions without judgment. Dialectics help us accept the contradictions in emotions and increase flexibility. This flexibility helps us understand our own and our loved one's experiences. What do you think about this process for Making Meaning?

Using Reflection to Find Meaning

Next you will guide the dyad in a reflection exercise focused on the patient, the caregiver, and their relationship. You will not have time to go over all the questions on page 76 of the Workbook, so select the most relevant questions based on your knowledge of the dyad—or let them pick. Make sure there is time to reflect on questions for the patient, the caregiver, and the relationship. Try to spend about 5 minutes per question and pick about three. You can consider asking the same questions for the patient and caregiver, if appropriate.

Turn to page 76 in your Workbook. We will use reflection to find meaning. We will pick from questions in the patient, caregiver, and relationship categories.

What do you wish people could understand about your experience during and after the acute brain illness? What is something in your life that you have gained since the ANI?

How has your perspective on your relationship changed?

If the dyad members have a hard time with this exercise including seeing positive aspects of the ANI, guide them using examples from prior sessions or your own observations. For example:

I remember the first time we discussed communication skills and how challenging that was. How do you think you are communicating now?

Encourage the dyad to review the Making Meaning Explainer Video by searching for this book's title on the Oxford Academic platform at academic.oup.com.

Using Mindfulness to Find Meaning

This section of the Clinician Guide provides a concise treatment course that the dyad can take with them after the program ends. Reviewing Mindful Stoplight, Dialectics, and Acceptance and Change will help summarize the work in a way that assists with termination. These skills are related to the concept of Making Meaning and are also included to ensure that the dyad can continue using them after the end of treatment.

Mindfulness can be helpful in Making Meaning. Mindfulness slows us down so that we can Observe, Describe, and Act with Awareness. How might you be able to use mindfulness to find meaning?

Ask the dyad members to use the Mindful Stoplight to reflect on thoughts, feelings, and behaviors. If they have trouble, use the examples in the Workbook.

Dialectics

Dialectics can also help us find meaning and sort through contradictions that come up after challenging experiences. Since the ANI, you and your loved one have faced challenging moments. Perhaps someone you care about disappointed you or said something hurtful. And someone else, at the same time, listened and helped you cope. Can you think of some Dialectics, and how you might sort through them?

If helpful, point the dyad to the figure on page 77 in the Workbook. Discuss how Dialectics are like puzzle pieces that we need to sort through and put together. Reinforce that acknowledging Dialectics helps us see the bigger picture without struggling with thoughts and feelings. Rather than choosing one thought, we can accept that there are multiple truths, multiple perspectives, and multiple experiences.

On page 77 of your Workbooks, we see puzzle pieces with contradictions that can fit together into a cohesive story. Can you think about some pieces of a puzzle of your own story as patient, caregiver, and together?

Acceptance and Change

Remind the dyad about the skill of Acceptance and Change (Dialectics). Discuss how to use acceptance to reflect, and how to help each other communicate about changes.

Acceptance helps us tolerate things we cannot control. Because many things after an ANI are outside of your control, you've likely been using acceptance throughout the journey. You can practice acceptance through Deep Breathing, Mindful Stoplight, and Dialectics. You can use the examples from the Workbook on pages 77–78.

At the same time, there are some things that we CAN change by communicating with our partner or by the behaviors we choose. On pages 77–78 of the Workbook there are some examples. Can you think of others to add?

Orient the patient and caregiver to the summary and table of skills at the end of Session 7 in the Workbook. Briefly review the session content and skills and ask them when skill(s) may be helpful to use.

Turn to page 78 in your Workbooks to review a summary of our session. Today, we discussed Making Meaning and reviewed other program skills. What skills do you think you will continue using?

Share with the dyad that you think they have the skills and tools they need to continue forward successfully in their recovery and that you believe in their shared mission for healing post-ANI.

Comment on their progress and your appraisal of their specific emotional distress remission (if applicable). It may be helpful to present how their scores on HADS and PCL improved over time (from first session to last). Express gratitude to the patient and caregiver for the work you have completed together during this program, and express confidence that they will continue being successful in their recovery journey.

The end of treatment will look different for each dyad based on the therapeutic relationship. Leave plenty of time for the dyad members and yourself to process the ending of services. Speak with your supervisor or colleagues about any difficulties you have.

Prescription for Recovery (Home Practice)

Remind the dyad about the weekly Prescription for Recovery section. Ask for specific times that they will plan to use the skills even after the program ends.

I encourage you to practice these skills alone and together from now on. And remember that the website can facilitate practice. We created recordings that can be accessed by searching for this book's title on the Oxford Academic platform at academic.oup.com. Make note of when you use them and if/how they are helpful.

Thank the dyad for their engagement in the program. Answer any final questions. If you are comfortable doing so, encourage them to reach out in the future if needed.

Thank you for your engagement in the program! Any final questions? I very much enjoyed working together and I wish you the best of luck! Reach out if you need more help.

References

Adhikari, N. K. J., Tansey, C. M., McAndrews, M. P., Matté, A., Pinto, R., Cheung, A. M., Diaz-Granados, N., & Herridge, M. S. (2011). Self-reported depressive symptoms and memory complaints in survivors five years after ARDS. *Chest*, *140*(6), 1484–1493. https://doi.org/10.1378/chest.11-1667

Ayerbe, L., Ayis, S., Wolfe, C. D. A., & Rudd, A. G. (2013). Natural history, predictors and outcomes of depression after stroke: Systematic review and meta-analysis. *British Journal of Psychiatry*, *202*(1), 14–21. https://doi.org/10.1192/bjp.bp.111.107664

Bannon, S., Lester, E. G., Gates, M. V., McCurley, J., Lin, A., Rosand, J., & Vranceanu, A.-M. (2020). Recovering Together: Building resiliency in dyads of stroke patients and their caregivers at risk for chronic emotional distress; a feasibility study. *Pilot and Feasibility Studies*, *6*(1), 75. https://doi.org/10.1186/s40814-020-00615-z

Bannon, S. M., Cornelius, T., Gates, M. V., Lester, E., Mace, R. A., Popok, P., Macklin, E. A., Rosand, J., & Vranceanu, A.-M. (2022). Emotional distress in neuro-ICU survivor–caregiver dyads: The Recovering Together randomized clinical trial. *Health Psychology*, *41*(4), 268–277. https://doi.org/10.1037/hea0001102

Barclay-Goddard, R., King, J., Dubouloz, C.-J., & Schwartz, C. E. (2012). Building on transformative learning and response shift theory to investigate health-related quality of life changes over time in individuals with chronic health conditions and disability. *Archives of Physical Medicine and Rehabilitation*, *93*(2), 214–220. https://doi.org/10.1016/j.apmr.2011.09.010

Barr, J., Fraser, G. L., Puntillo, K., Ely, E. W., Gélinas, C., Dasta, J. F., Davidson, J. E., Devlin, J. W., Kress, J. P., Joffe, A. M., Coursin, D. B., Herr, D. L., Tung, A., Robinson, B. R. H., Fontaine, D. K., Ramsay, M. A., Riker, R. R., Sessler, C. N., Pun, B., . . . American College of Critical Care Medicine. (2013). Clinical practice guidelines for the management of pain, agitation, and delirium in adult patients in the intensive care unit. *Critical Care Medicine*, *41*(1), 263–306. https://doi.org/10.1097/CCM.0b013e3182783b72

Barreto, B. B., Luz, M., Rios, M. N. D. O., Lopes, A. A., & Gusmao-Flores, D. (2019). The impact of intensive care unit diaries on patients' and relatives' outcomes: A systematic review and meta-analysis. *Critical Care, 23*(1), 411. https://doi.org/10.1186/s13054-019-2678-0

Blevins, C. A., Weathers, F. W., Davis, M. T., Witte, T. K., & Domino, J. L. (2015). The Posttraumatic Stress Disorder Checklist for *DSM-5* (PCL-5): Development and initial psychometric evaluation. *Journal of Traumatic Stress, 28*(6), 489–498. https://doi.org/10.1002/jts.22059

Bodenmann, G., Falconier, M. K., & Randall, A. K. (2019). Editorial: Dyadic coping. *Frontiers in Psychology, 10.* https://www.frontiersin.org/articles/10.3389/fpsyg.2019.01498

Choi, J., Donahoe, M. P., & Hoffman, L. A. (2016). Psychological and physical health in family caregivers of intensive care unit survivors: Current knowledge and future research strategies. *Journal of Korean Academy of Nursing, 46*(2), 159–167. https://doi.org/10.4040/jkan.2016.46.2.159

Choi, K. W., Shaffer, K. M., Zale, E. L., Funes, C. J., Koenen, K. C., Tehan, T., Rosand, J., & Vranceanu, A.-M. (2018). Early risk and resiliency factors predict chronic posttraumatic stress disorder in caregivers of patients admitted to a neuroscience ICU. *Critical Care Medicine, 46*(5), 713–719. https://doi.org/10.1097/CCM.0000000000002988

Chung, C. R., Yoo, H. J., Park, J., & Ryu, S. (2017). Cognitive impairment and psychological distress at discharge from intensive care unit. *Psychiatry Investigation, 14*(3), 376–379. https://doi.org/10.4306/pi.2017.14.3.376

Cook, W. L., & Kenny, D. A. (2005). The actor–partner interdependence model: A model of bidirectional effects in developmental studies. *International Journal of Behavioral Development, 29*(2), 101–109. https://doi.org/10.1080/01650250444000405

Davydow, D. S., Hough, C. L., Langa, K. M., & Iwashyna, T. J. (2012). Depressive symptoms in spouses of older patients with severe sepsis. *Critical Care Medicine, 40*(8), 2335–2341. https://doi.org/10.1097/CCM.0b013e3182536a81

Denno, M. S., Gillard, P. J., Graham, G. D., DiBonaventura, M. D., Goren, A., Varon, S. F., & Zorowitz, R. (2013). Anxiety and depression associated with caregiver burden in caregivers of stroke survivors with spasticity. *Archives of Physical Medicine and Rehabilitation, 94*(9), 1731–1736. https://doi.org/10.1016/j.apmr.2013.03.014

Devlin, J. W., & Roberts, R. J. (2009). Pharmacology of commonly used analgesics and sedatives in the ICU: Benzodiazepines, propofol, and opioids. *Critical Care Clinics, 25*(3), 431–449. https://doi.org/10.1016/j.ccc.2009.03.003

Fraser, G. L., Devlin, J. W., Worby, C. P., Alhazzani, W., Barr, J., Dasta, J. F., Kress, J. P., Davidson, J. E., & Spencer, F. A. (2013). Benzodiazepine versus nonbenzodiazepine-based sedation for mechanically ventilated, critically ill adults: A systematic review and meta-analysis of randomized trials. *Critical Care Medicine*, *41*(9 Suppl 1), S30–S38. https://doi.org/10.1097/CCM.0b013e3182a16898

Gries, C. J., Engelberg, R. A., Kross, E. K., Zatzick, D., Nielsen, E. L., Downey, L., & Curtis, J. R. (2010). Predictors of symptoms of posttraumatic stress and depression in family members after patient death in the ICU. *Chest*, *137*(2), 280–287. https://doi.org/10.1378/chest.09-1291

Hammond, F. M., Barrett, R. S., Shea, T., Seel, R. T., McAlister, T. W., Kaelin, D., Ryser, D., Corrigan, J. D., Cullen, N., & Horn, S. D. (2015). Psychotropic medication use during inpatient rehabilitation for traumatic brain injury. *Archives of Physical Medicine and Rehabilitation*, *96*(8 Suppl), S256–S273. https://doi.org/10.1016/j.apmr.2015.01.025

Hirtz, D., Thurman, D. J., Gwinn-Hardy, K., Mohamed, M., Chaudhuri, A. R., & Zalutsky, R. (2007). How common are the "common" neurologic disorders? *Neurology*, *68*(5), 326–337. https://doi.org/10.1212/01.wnl.0000252807.38124.a3

Hopkins, R. O., Key, C. W., Suchyta, M. R., Weaver, L. K., & Orme, J. F. (2010). Risk factors for depression and anxiety in survivors of acute respiratory distress syndrome. *General Hospital Psychiatry*, *32*(2), 147–155. https://doi.org/10.1016/j.genhosppsych.2009.11.003

Jackson, J. C., Archer, K. R., Bauer, R., Abraham, C. M., Song, Y., Greevey, R., Guillamondegui, O., Ely, E. W., & Obremskey, W. (2011). A prospective investigation of long-term cognitive impairment and psychological distress in moderately versus severely injured trauma intensive care unit survivors without intracranial hemorrhage. *Journal of Trauma*, *71*(4), 860–866. https://doi.org/10.1097/TA.0b013e3182151961

Jackson, J. C., Pandharipande, P. P., Girard, T. D., Brummel, N. E., Thompson, J. L., Hughes, C. G., Pun, B. T., Vasilevskis, E. E., Morandi, A., Shintani, A. K., Hopkins, R. O., Bernard, G. R., Dittus, R. S., Ely, E. W., & Bringing to Light the Risk Factors and Incidence of Neuropsychological Dysfunction in ICU Survivors (BRAIN-ICU) study investigators. (2014). Depression, post-traumatic stress disorder, and functional disability in survivors of critical illness in the BRAIN-ICU study: A longitudinal cohort study. *Lancet Respiratory Medicine*, *2*(5), 369–379. https://doi.org/10.1016/S2213-2600(14)70051-7

Kabat-Zinn, J. (2003). Mindfulness-based interventions in context: Past, present, and future. *Clinical Psychology: Science and Practice, 10*(2), 144–156. https://doi.org/10.1093/clipsy.bpg016

Kelly, J. M., Rubenfeld, G. D., Masson, N., Min, A., & Adhikari, N. K. J. (2017). Using selective serotonin reuptake inhibitors and serotonin-norepinephrine reuptake inhibitors in critical care: A systematic review of the evidence for benefit or harm. *Critical Care Medicine, 45*(6), e607–e616. https://doi.org/10.1097/CCM.0000000000002308

Kessler, R. C., Chiu, W. T., Demler, O., Merikangas, K. R., & Walters, E. E. (2005). Prevalence, severity, and comorbidity of 12-month DSM-IV disorders in the National Comorbidity Survey Replication. *Archives of General Psychiatry, 62*(6), 617–627. https://doi.org/10.1001/archpsyc.62.6.617

Linehan, M. M., & Wilks, C. R. (2015). The course and evolution of dialectical behavior therapy. *American Journal of Psychotherapy, 69*(2), 97–110. https://doi.org/10.1176/appi.psychotherapy.2015.69.2.97

May, J. M., Richardi, T. M., & Barth, K. S. (2016). Dialectical behavior therapy as treatment for borderline personality disorder. *Mental Health Clinician, 6*(2), 62–67. https://doi.org/10.9740/mhc.2016.03.62

McCurley, J. L., Funes, C. J., Zale, E. L., Lin, A., Jacobo, M., Jacobs, J. M., Salgueiro, D., Tehan, T., Rosand, J., & Vranceanu, A.-M. (2019). Preventing chronic emotional distress in stroke survivors and their informal caregivers. *Neurocritical Care, 30*(3), 581–589. https://doi.org/10.1007/s12028-018-0641-6

Meyers, E. E., McCurley, J., Lester, E., Jacobo, M., Rosand, J., & Vranceanu, A.-M. (2020). Building resiliency in dyads of patients admitted to the neuroscience intensive care unit and their family caregivers: Lessons learned from William and Laura. *Cognitive and Behavioral Practice, 27*(3), 321–335. https://doi.org/10.1016/j.cbpra.2020.02.001

Mikkelsen, M. E., Christie, J. D., Lanken, P. N., Biester, R. C., Thompson, B. T., Bellamy, S. L., Localio, A. R., Demissie, E., Hopkins, R. O., & Angus, D. C. (2012). The Adult Respiratory Distress Syndrome Cognitive Outcomes Study. *American Journal of Respiratory and Critical Care Medicine, 185*(12), 1307–1315. https://doi.org/10.1164/rccm.201111-2025OC

Myhren, H., Ekeberg, O., Tøien, K., Karlsson, S., & Stokland, O. (2010). Posttraumatic stress, anxiety and depression symptoms in patients during the first year post intensive care unit discharge. *Critical Care (London, England), 14*(1), R14. https://doi.org/10.1186/cc8870

Paparrigopoulos, T., Melissaki, A., Tzavellas, E., Karaiskos, D., Ilias, I., & Kokras, N. (2014). Increased co-morbidity of depression and post-traumatic stress disorder symptoms and common risk factors in intensive care unit survivors: A two-year follow-up study. *International Journal of Psychiatry in Clinical Practice*, *18*(1), 25–31. https://doi.org/10.3109/13651501.2013.855793

Parker, A. M., Sricharoenchai, T., Raparla, S., Schneck, K. W., Bienvenu, O. J., & Needham, D. M. (2015). Posttraumatic stress disorder in critical illness survivors: A meta-analysis. *Critical Care Medicine*, *43*(5), 1121–1129. https://doi.org/10.1097/CCM.0000000000000882

Petrinec, A. B., & Martin, B. R. (2018). Post-intensive care syndrome symptoms and health-related quality of life in family decision-makers of critically ill patients. *Palliative & Supportive Care*, *16*(6), 719–724. https://doi.org/10.1017/S1478951517001043

Rizvi, S. L., Steffel, L. M., & Carson-Wong, A. (2013). An overview of dialectical behavior therapy for professional psychologists. *Professional Psychology: Research and Practice*, *44*(2), 73–80. https://doi.org/10.1037/a0029808

Shafiekhani, M., Mirjalili, M., & Vazin, A. (2018). Psychotropic drug therapy in patients in the intensive care unit—usage, adverse effects, and drug interactions: A review. *Therapeutics and Clinical Risk Management*, *14*, 1799–1812. https://doi.org/10.2147/TCRM.S176079

Shields, C. G., King, D. A., & Wynne, L. C. (1995). Interventions with later life families. In R. H. Mikesell, D.-D. Lusterman, & S. H. McDaniel (Eds.), *Integrating family therapy: Handbook of family psychology and systems theory* (pp. 141–158). American Psychological Association. https://doi.org/10.1037/10172-008

Siegel, M. D., Hayes, E., Vanderwerker, L. C., Loseth, D. B., & Prigerson, H. G. (2008). Psychiatric illness in the next of kin of patients who die in the intensive care unit. *Critical Care Medicine*, *36*(6), 1722–1728. https://doi.org/10.1097/CCM.0b013e318174da72

Southwick, S. M., Bonanno, G. A., Masten, A. S., Panter-Brick, C., & Yehuda, R. (2014). Resilience definitions, theory, and challenges: Interdisciplinary perspectives. *European Journal of Psychotraumatology*, *5*(1), 25338. https://doi.org/10.3402/ejpt.v5.25338

Thomason, J. W. W., Shintani, A., Peterson, J. F., Pun, B. T., Jackson, J. C., & Ely, E. W. (2005). Intensive care unit delirium is an independent predictor of longer hospital stay: A prospective analysis of 261 non-ventilated patients. *Critical Care (London, England)*, *9*(4), R375–381. https://doi.org/10.1186/cc3729

van Beusekom, I., Bakhshi-Raiez, F., de Keizer, N. F., Dongelmans, D. A., & van der Schaaf, M. (2016). Reported burden on informal caregivers of ICU survivors: A literature review. *Critical Care (London, England)*, *20*, 16. https://doi.org/10.1186/s13054-016-1185-9

van den Born-van Zanten, S. A., Dongelmans, D. A., Dettling-Ihnenfeldt, D., Vink, R., & van der Schaaf, M. (2016). Caregiver strain and posttraumatic stress symptoms of informal caregivers of intensive care unit survivors. *Rehabilitation Psychology*, *61*(2), 173–178. https://doi.org/10.1037/rep0000081

Vehviläinen, J., Skrifvars, M. B., Reinikainen, M., Bendel, S., Marinkovic, I., Ala-Kokko, T., Hoppu, S., Laitio, R., Siironen, J., & Raj, R. (2021). Psychotropic medication use among patients with a traumatic brain injury treated in the intensive care unit: A multi-centre observational study. *Acta Neurochirurgica*, *163*(10), 2909–2917. https://doi.org/10.1007/s00701-021-04956-3

Vranceanu, A.-M., Bannon, S., Mace, R., Lester, E., Meyers, E., Gates, M., Popok, P., Lin, A., Salgueiro, D., Tehan, T., Macklin, E., & Rosand, J. (2020). Feasibility and efficacy of a resiliency intervention for the prevention of chronic emotional distress among survivor–caregiver dyads admitted to the neuroscience intensive care unit: A randomized clinical trial. *JAMA Network Open*, *3*(10), e2020807. https://doi.org/10.1001/jamanetworkopen.2020.20807

Vranceanu, A.-M., Woodworth, E. C., Kanaya, M. R., Bannon, S., Mace, R. A., Manglani, H., Duarte, B. A., Rush, C. L., Choukas, N. R., Briskin, E. A., Cohen, J., Parker, R., Macklin, E., Lester, E., Traeger, L., Rosand, J., Grunberg, V. A., Qualls, S. R., Kowal, C., . . . Konner, K. M. (2022). The Recovering Together study protocol: A single-blind RCT to prevent chronic emotional distress in patient-caregiver dyads in the Neuro-ICU. *Contemporary Clinical Trials*, *123*, 106998. https://doi.org/10.1016/j.cct.2022.106998

Wade, D. M., Mouncey, P. R., Richards-Belle, A., Wulff, J., Harrison, D. A., Sadique, M. Z., Grieve, R. D., Emerson, L. M., Mason, A. J., Aaronovitch, D., Als, N., Brewin, C. R., Harvey, S. E., Howell, D. C. J., Hudson, N., Mythen, M. G., Smyth, D., Weinman, J., Welch, J., . . . for the POPPI Trial Investigators. (2019). Effect of a nurse-led preventive psychological intervention on symptoms of posttraumatic stress disorder among critically ill patients: A randomized clinical trial. *JAMA*, *321*(7), 665. https://doi.org/10.1001/jama.2019.0073

White, D. B., Cua, S. M., Walk, R., Pollice, L., Weissfeld, L., Hong, S., Landefeld, C. S., & Arnold, R. M. (2012). Nurse-led intervention to improve surrogate decision making for patients with advanced critical illness. *American Journal of Critical Care*, *21*(6), 396–409. https://doi.org/10.4037/ajcc2012223

Wintermann, G.-B., Weidner, K., Strauß, B., Rosendahl, J., & Petrowski, K. (2016). Predictors of posttraumatic stress and quality of life in family members of chronically critically ill patients after intensive care. *Annals of Intensive Care, 6*, 69. https://doi.org/10.1186/s13613-016-0174-0

Yehuda, R. (2002). Post-traumatic stress disorder. *New England Journal of Medicine, 346*(2), 108–114. https://doi.org/10.1056/NEJMra012941

Zigmond, A. S., & Snaith, R. P. (1983). The Hospital Anxiety and Depression Scale. *Acta Psychiatrica Scandinavica, 67*(6), 361–370. https://doi.org/10.1111/j.1600-0447.1983.tb09716.x

Zimmerli, M., Tisljar, K., Balestra, G.-M., Langewitz, W., Marsch, S., & Hunziker, S. (2014). Prevalence and risk factors for post-traumatic stress disorder in relatives of out-of-hospital cardiac arrest patients. *Resuscitation, 85*(6), 801–808. https://doi.org/10.1016/j.resuscitation.2014.02.022